VMS

VISUAL MNEMONICS FOR MICROBIOLOGY AND IMMUNOLOGY

VMS

VISUAL MNEMONICS FOR MICROBIOLOGY AND IMMUNOLOGY

LAURIE L. MARBAS
Texas Tech University Health Sciences Center
Class of 2003
School of Medicine
Lubbock, Texas

JOHN W. PELLEY, PHD
Associate Professor in Cell Biology and Biochemistry
Texas Tech University HSC
School of Medicine
Lubbock, Texas

Blackwell
Science

Editorial Offices:
Commerce Place, 350 Main Street, Malden, Massachusetts 02148, USA
Osney Mead, Oxford OX2 0EL, England
25 John Street, London WC1N 2BS, England
23 Ainslie Place, Edinburgh EH3 6AJ, Scotland
54 University Street, Carlton, Victoria 3053, Australia

Other Editorial Offices:
Blackwell Wissenschafts-Verlag GmbH, Kurfürstendamm 57, 10707 Berlin, Germany
Blackwell Science KK, MG Kodenmacho Building, 7-10 Kodenmacho Nihombashi, Chuo-ku, Tokyo 104, Japan
Iowa State University Press, A Blackwell Science Company, 2121 S. State Avenue, Ames, Iowa 50014-8300, USA

Distributors:

The Americas
Blackwell Publishing
c/o AIDC
P.O. Box 20
50 Winter Sport Lane
Williston, VT 05495-0020
(Telephone orders: 800-216-2522; fax orders: 802-864-7626)

Australia
Blackwell Science Pty, Ltd.
54 University Street
Carlton, Victoria 3053
(Telephone orders: 03-9347-0300; fax orders: 03-9349-3016)

Outside The Americas and Australia
Blackwell Science, Ltd.
c/o Marston Book Services, Ltd.
P.O. Box 269
Abingdon
Oxon OX14 4YN
England
(Telephone orders: 44-01235-465500; fax orders: 44-01235-465555)

Acquisitions: Beverly Copland
Development: Julia Casson
Production: Shawn Girsberger
Manufacturing: Lisa Flanagan
Marketing Manager: Toni Fournier
Illustration remastering by Frank Habit
Cover design by Meral Dabcovich, Visual Perspectives
Interior design by Shawn Girsberger
Typeset by Software Services
Printed and bound by Sheridan Books

Printed in the United States of America
01 02 03 04 5 4 3 2 1

Library of Congress Cataloging-in-Publication Data

Marbas, Laurie L.
Visual mnemonics for microbiology and immunology / by Laurie L. Marbas, John W. Pelley.
p. ; cm.—(Visual mnemonics series)
ISBN 0-632-04587-6
1. Medical microbiology—Study and teaching. 2. Immunology—Study and teaching. 3. Mnemonics. I. Title. II. Series.
[DNLM: 1. Microbiology—Terminology—English. 2. Allergy and Immunology—Terminology—English. 3. Association Learning—Terminology—English. 4. Parasitology—Terminology—English. QW 15 M312v 2001]
QR46 .M4345 2001
616'.01'071—dc21 2001035415

CONTENTS

PREFACE

Visual Mnemonics for Microbiology and Immunology is a study tool that will help you to quickly learn and memorize material presented in Medical Microbiology. It is visual because much of our memory is created from images, and it is mnemonic because it is constructed to aid rapid recall on examinations. Two significant features of *Visual Mnemonics for Microbiology and Immunology* are the use of humor and exaggeration, both of which are well established as memory tools, and the use of connections as an aid to integrative learning. The results you can expect are long-term retention of material and an increased rate of learning. This allows you more time to study the remainder of the material that is not covered in the *Visual Mnemonics for Microbiology and Immunology* book.

These illustrations were created to assist in my own studying, because I was always short on time to efficiently memorize facts, and because I was frustrated when I couldn't remember them longer than the hour after the test. As a mother of three small children my time for studying is limited, and must be high yield 100% of the time. These illustrations allowed me to do that, and judging from their requests for copies, it worked for many of my classmates also. Several of them stated to me that their grades improved 10 points from one exam to the next largely due to the extra study time they had gained. Also, we all agree that the long-term retention from these illustrations is incredible compared to traditional study methods of memorizing from lists or note cards.

I have attempted to combine as many pertinent facts and functions into the illustrations as possible. This book is not meant to be a total solution to your studying, but it certainly can provide an efficient and more stimulating method of learning the material.

Here are some tips on using the pictures:

1. Look at them after you have read your class notes. This will reveal what material is deemed important in your particular curriculum and what might not be covered in these illustrations, but it won't be much.
2. Write on them, color them, redraw them, add your own drawings to them – the more these illustrations are manipulated and customized by you, the more information will be retained in long-term memory. We have provided space for you to do this.
3. Since most students rewrite notes while they study, you can also record this information in the book. It will be concise and everything will be in one place for you.

I am so happy I could share my notes with you. You're in control now, so now go ahead and learn!

ACKNOWLEDGMENTS

Throughout my medical education I have been blessed with many opportunities which I thank the Lord for everyday. A special thank you must go to my grandmother, Maxine Turner, for watching my three children while I attend school and without her none of this would have been possible. My husband, Patrick Marbas, is also deserving of a tremendous debt of gratitude for making many sacrifices for me, including driving 100 miles one-way to work everyday, so that I could attend medical school. In addition, much love to my three beautiful children, Emily, Jonathan, and Gabriel, for playing quietly while I study and giving me hugs of encouragement when I needed it the most.

Also, thank you to Dr. Pelley for not only helping me with this project, but also inspiring me with his learning and study methods. His insight enlightened me and brought forth many of the ideas incorporated into these illustrations. I would also like to say thank you to Dr. Jane Colmer-Hamood, Dr. David Straus, and Dr. Rial Rolfe for their support and encouragement.

Finally, I would like to thank Erin Case, Sheemain Asaria, Nehal Shah, and my mother, Patricia Lockridge, for their friendship and creative support throughout this project. Their encouragement has been invaluable and greatly appreciated.

CONSULTING ILLUSTRATORS

Erin Case
Texas Tech University School of Medicine
Class 2003

Nehal Shah
Texas Tech University School of Medicine
Class 2003

Sheemain Asaria
Texas Tech University School of Medicine
Class 2003

Patricia Lockridge

I.
PARASITOLOGY

NOTES

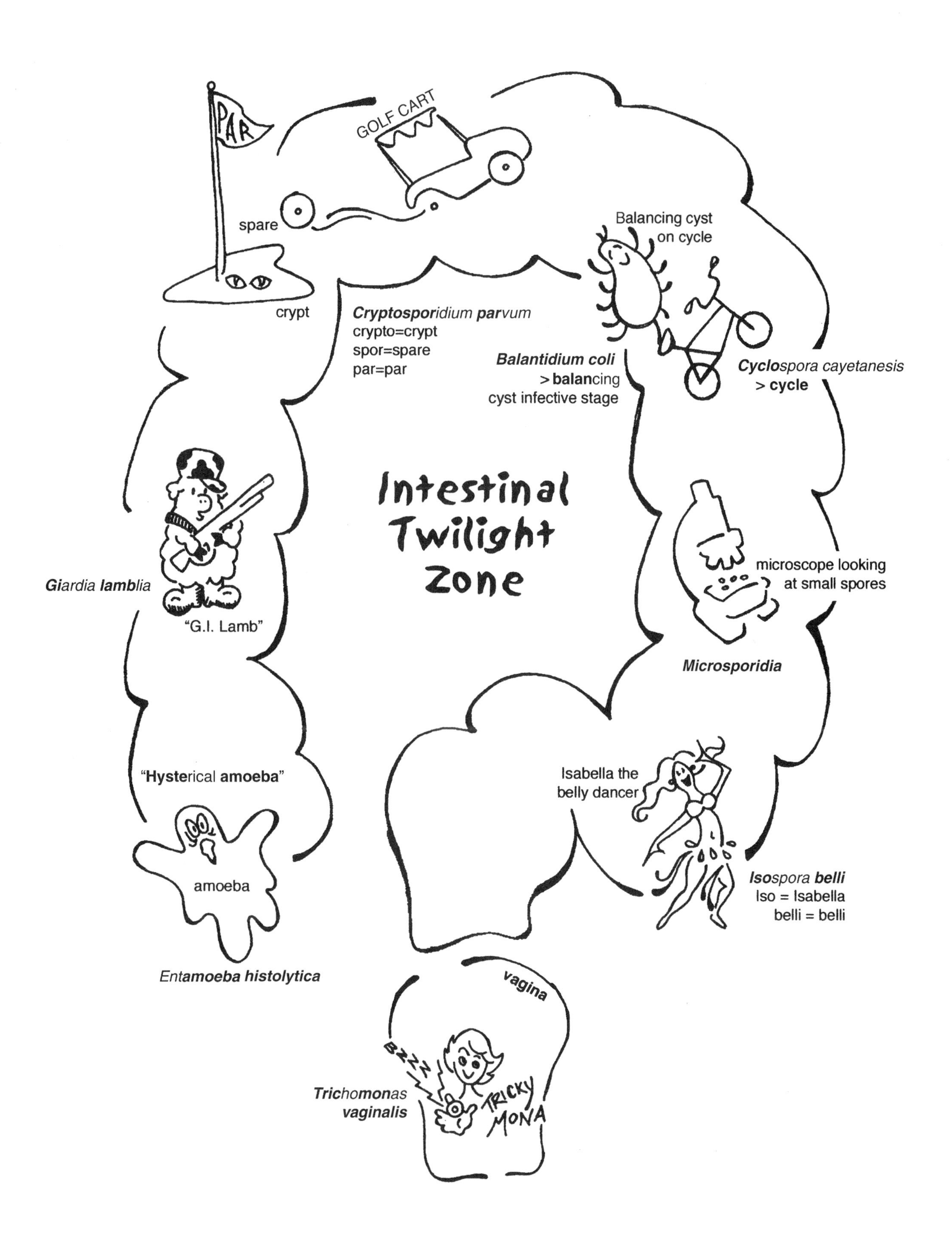
PAR
GOLF CART
spare
crypt
Cryptosporidium parvum
crypto=crypt
spor=spare
par=par
Balancing cyst
on cycle
Balantidium coli
> balancing
cyst infective stage
Cyclospora cayetanesis
> cycle
Intestinal
Twilight
Zone
Giardia lamblia
"G.I. Lamb"
microscope looking
at small spores
Microsporidia
"Hysterical amoeba"
amoeba
Entamoeba histolytica
Isabella the
belly dancer
Isospora belli
Iso = Isabella
belli = belli
vagina
BZZZ
TRICKY
MONA
Trichomonas
vaginalis

Hemoflagellates: RBC with Flagellum

NOTES

Cutaneous, Mucocutaneous, and Visceral Leishmaniasis ("leash on dog")

- biopsy beach
  - ⇒ diagnosis by biopsy
  - ⇒ sand fly transmit promastigote
- Donovan the Doberman
  - ⇒ visceral leishmaniasis ("Vic Leishman") caused by *Leishmania donovani*
  - ⇒ dog best reservoir ("doberman")
- treatment of amastigotes ("A" mast) with sodium gluconate
  - ⇒ sodium is the NA on the boat's sails
  - ⇒ gluconate is the G at the base of the boat

African Trypanosomiasis

⇒ a.k.a. African Sleeping Sickness
  - ⇒ "Africa and goes to sleep"
- trypomastigotes infective in tsetse fly
  - ⇒ Mr. T flies
- parasitemia and fever occur in waves
- Western African Sleeping Sickness
  - ⇒ humans are reservoir (*T. brucei gambiense*)
- Eastern African Sleeping Sickness
  - ⇒ **zoo**nosis (*T. brucei rhodesiense*)
    - ⇒ ("zoo")

Chagas' Disease

⇒ "chuga, chuga"
- American trypanosomiasis
  - ⇒ Americans
  - ⇒ Try Pan Some
- caused by *T. cruzi*
  - ⇒ Tom Cruzi
- **red**uviid **bug**'s (kissing bug) feces is vector
  - ⇒ red bug and feces
- Romana's Sign
  - ⇒ Romana

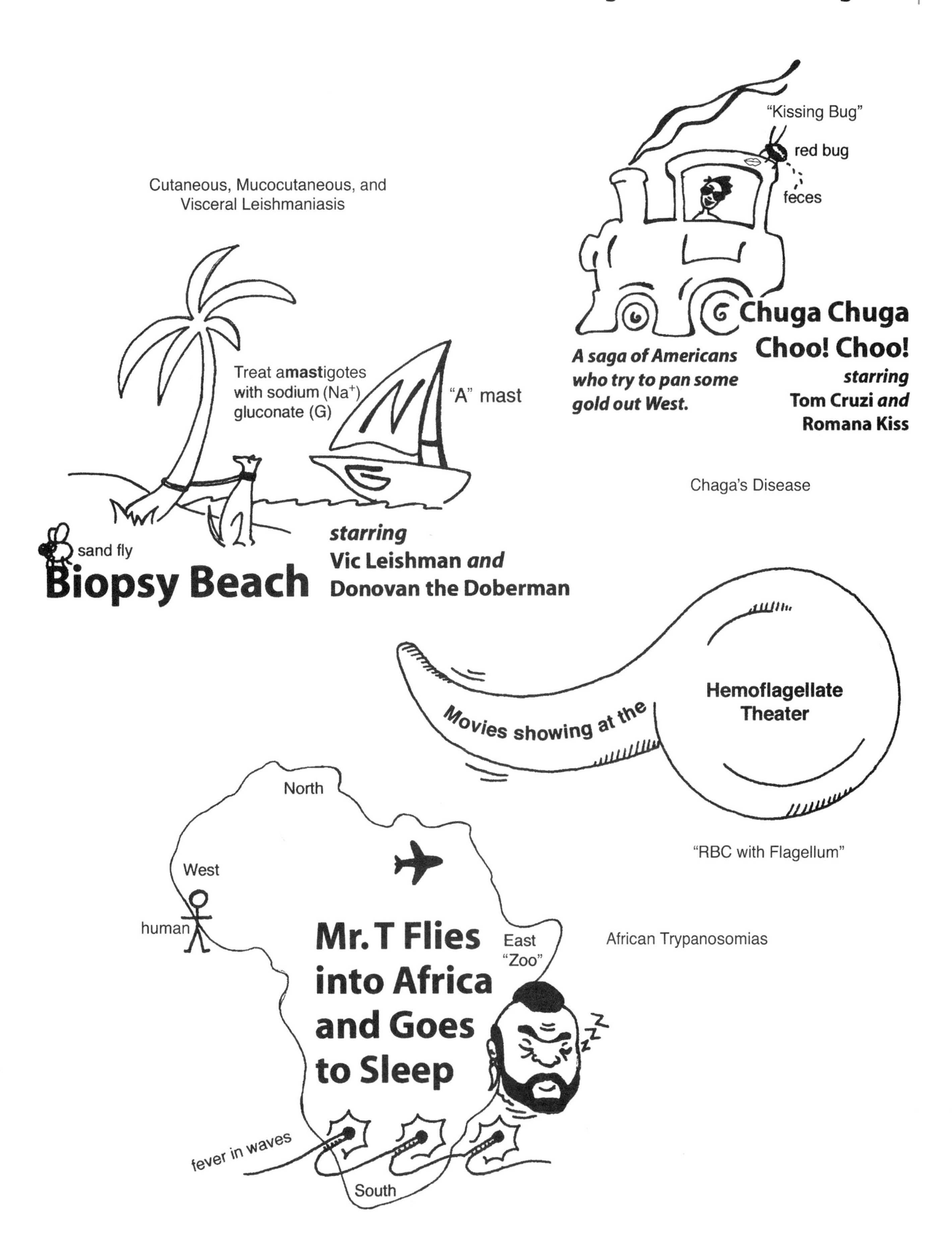
"Kissing Bug"
red bug
feces
Cutaneous, Mucocutaneous, and
Visceral Leishmaniasis
Chuga Chuga
Choo! Choo!
A saga of Americans
who try to pan some
gold out West.
starring
Tom Cruzi and
Romana Kiss
Treat amastigotes
with sodium (Na+)
gluconate (G)
"A" mast
Chaga's Disease
sand fly
Biopsy Beach
starring
Vic Leishman and
Donovan the Doberman
Movies showing at the
Hemoflagellate
Theater
North
"RBC with Flagellum"
West
human
Mr. T Flies
into Africa
and Goes
to Sleep
East
"Zoo"
African Trypanosomias
fever in waves
South

NOTES

- *Plasmodium vivax* ("VIVA") and *Plasmodium ovale* ("ovale") produce latent forms hypnozoites ("hypnotized zoite") in the liver which is responsible for relapses.

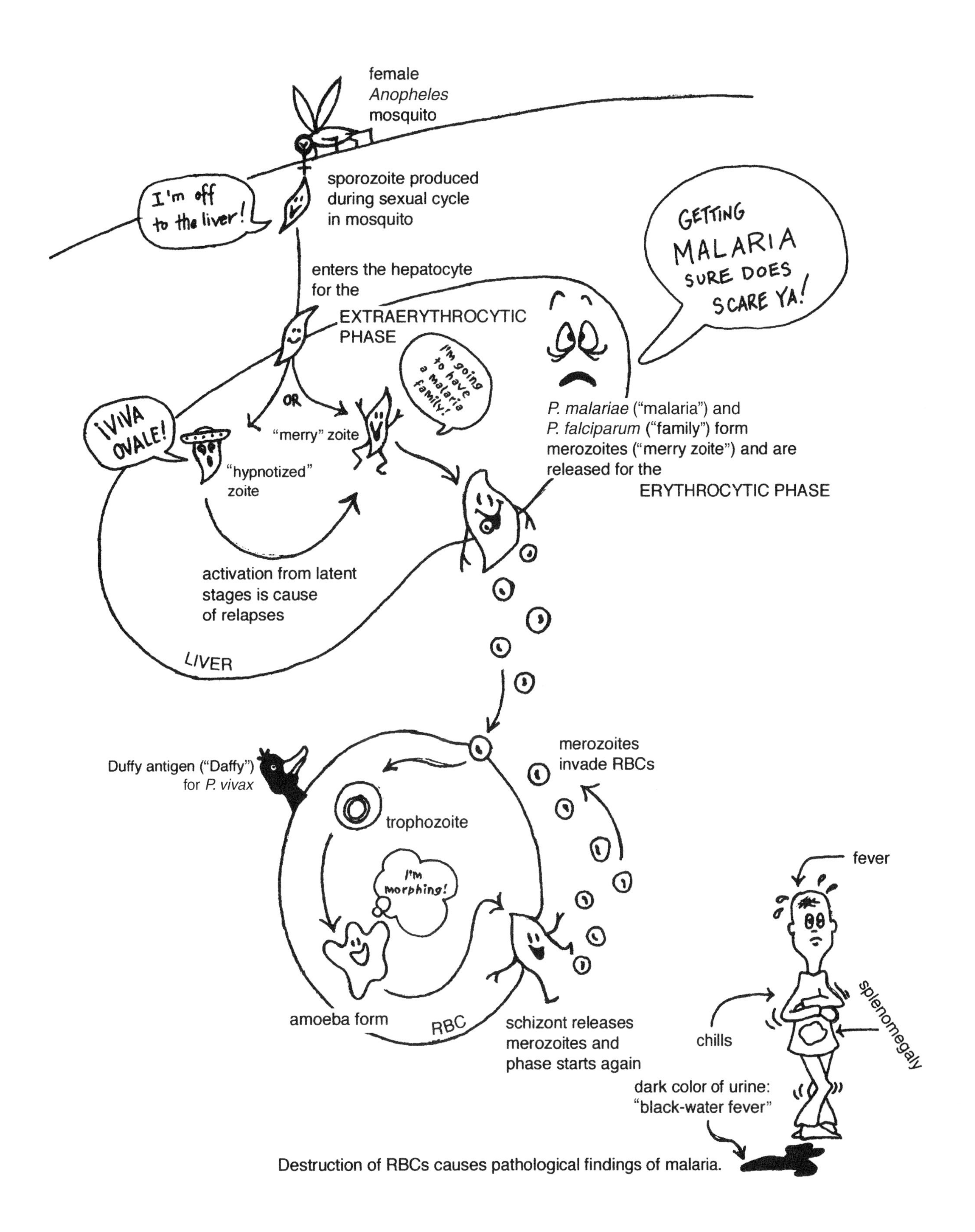

Destruction of RBCs causes pathological findings of malaria.

NOTES

Toxoplasmosis

⇒ ("toxic")

- caused by *Toxoplasma gondii* (cat name)
- transmission:
  - ⇒ trophozoites (trophy)→found in raw meat, transplacenta, transfusion
- oocytes (poocyte)→cat feces (gato is Spanish for cat)
- parasites block phagosome-lysosome fusion
- treat with pyrimethamine/trisulfapyrimidine

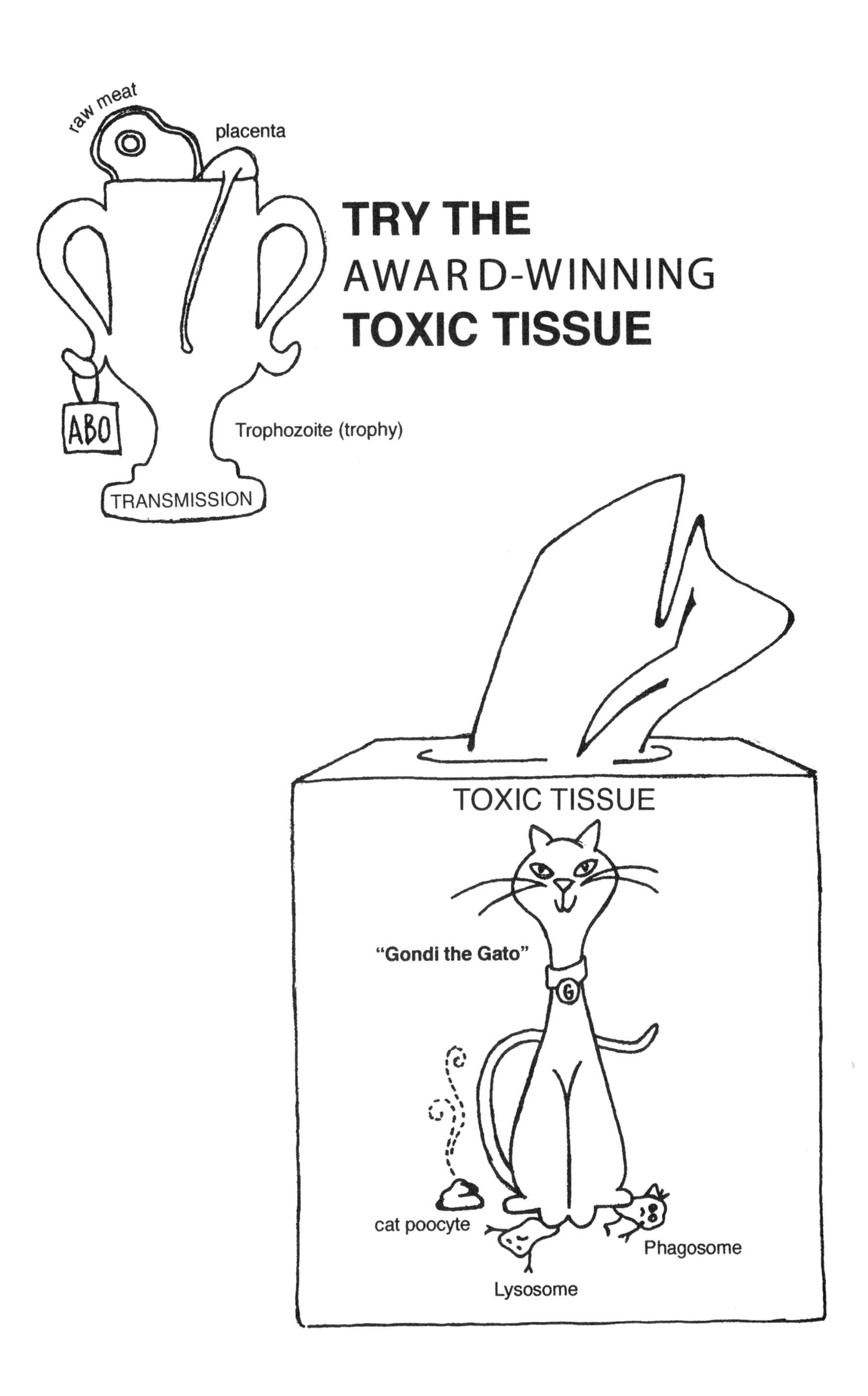
raw meat
placenta
TRY THE
AWARD-WINNING
TOXIC TISSUE
ABO
Trophozoite (trophy)
TRANSMISSION
TOXIC TISSUE
"Gondi the Gato"
G
cat poocyte
Phagosome
Lysosome

Trematodes (Flukes): Trim Toes

NOTES

Schistosoma—blood flukes
Clonorchis sinensis—liver flukes
Paragonimus westermani—lung flukes

Schistosomiasis (blood fluke)

⇒ SCHIZO LUKE
- infection by penetration of skin by **cerc**ariae⇒Capt. **Cerc**
- asexual reproduction in **snail**⇒escargot
- adults persist by immunologic **camouflage**
  ⇒ (camouflage outfits)
- eggs are pathogenic in gut or bladder
  ⇒ pregnant worm
- liver, spleen, lungs, and brain infected by metastasis
- causes bloody diarrhea and hematuria
- treatment with praziquantel
  ⇒ Prazi the Piranha

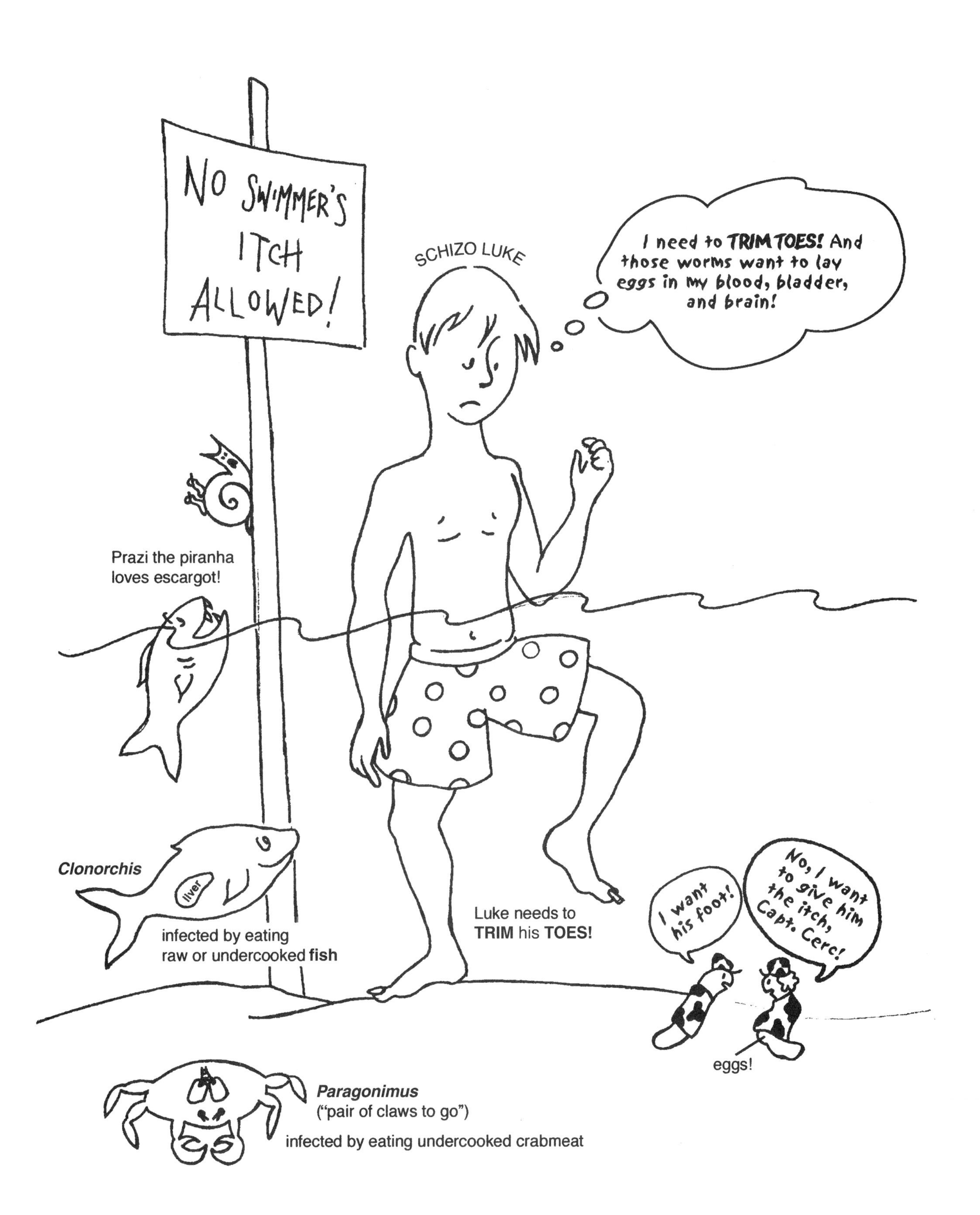
NO SWIMMER'S ITCH ALLOWED!
SCHIZO LUKE
I need to TRIM TOES! And those worms want to lay eggs in my blood, bladder, and brain!
Prazi the piranha loves escargot!
Clonorchis
liver
infected by eating raw or undercooked **fish**
Luke needs to **TRIM** his **TOES!**
I want his foot!
No, I want to give him the itch, Capt. Cerc!
eggs!
Paragonimus
("pair of claws to go")
infected by eating undercooked crabmeat

NOTES

Cysticercosis

⇒ cysts

- large (macroscopic) so can be seen with naked eye
- somatic infection which begins with a larval tapeworm
- any tissue involvement but primarily subcutaneous tissue, muscle, and brain
- form space-occupying lesions which are encased by inflammatory response
- treat with albendazole if symptomatic

Taeniasis

⇒ tiny taeniasis

- intestinal infection with adult tapeworm for which humans are only host
- cattle and pigs are reservoirs
- infection occurs by ingesting poorly cooked beef and pork

Hymenolepiasis

⇒ ("Dwarf rat must hide from men.")

- dwarf and rat tapeworm
- adult tapeworms confined to intestine
- internal autoinfection
- treat with praziquantel

Diphyllobothriasis

⇒ Phyllis × 2

- plerocercoid larvae infective
- infection occurs after ingestion of under-cooked fish
- small intestine only site of infection
- compete with host for B-12
- treat with praziquantel (Prazi the Piranha)

Echinococcus

⇒ Echinodermata is phylum of starfish
⇒ Coccus (rounded ends of starfish's arms)

- causes hydatid disease
  ⇒ High Do
- large cysts form

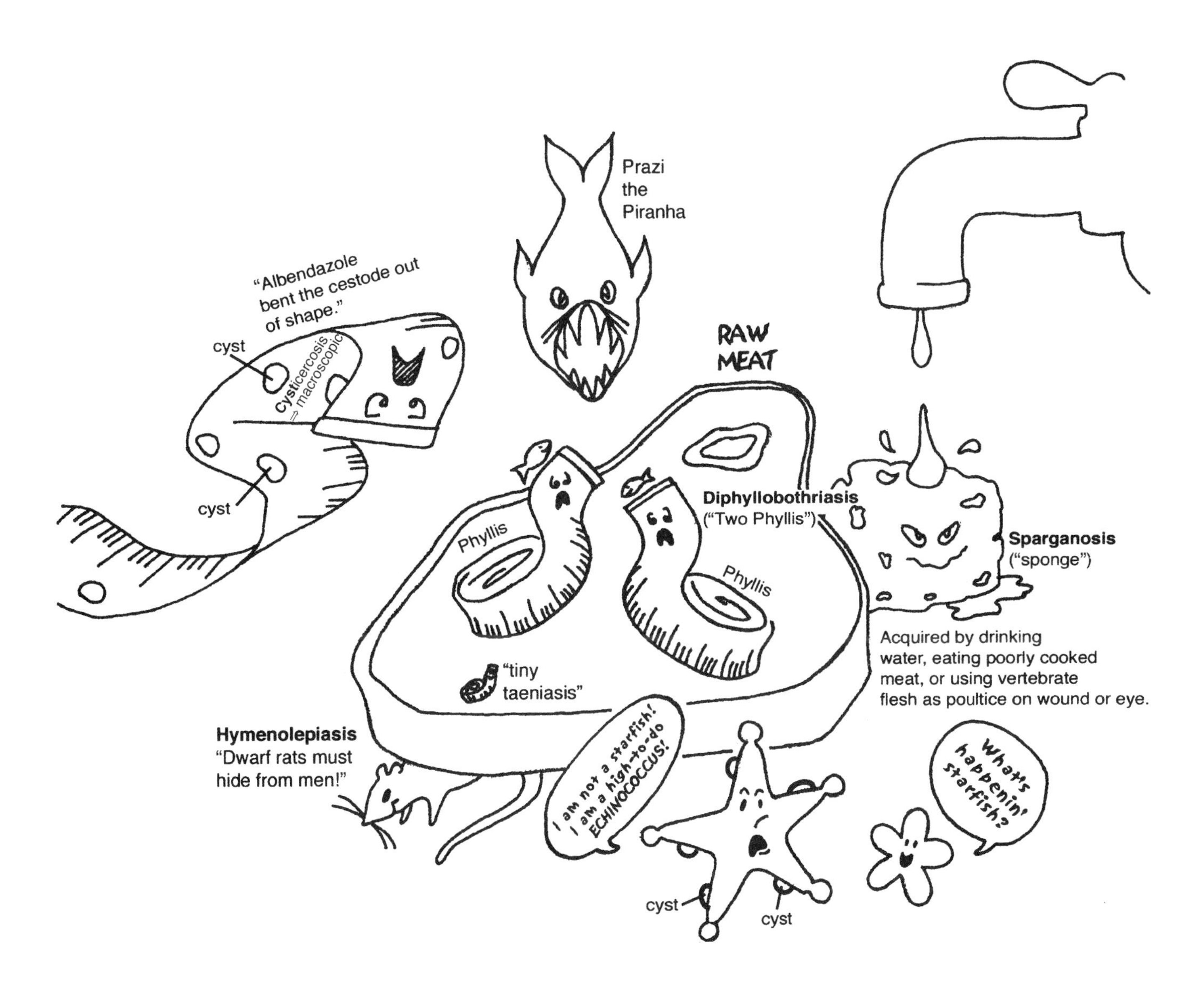
Prazi
the
Piranha
"Albendazole
bent the cestode out
of shape."
cyst
cysticercosis
⇒ macroscopic
cyst
RAW
MEAT
Diphyllobothriasis
("Two Phyllis")
Phyllis
Phyllis
Sparganosis
("sponge")
Acquired by drinking
water, eating poorly cooked
meat, or using vertebrate
flesh as poultice on wound or eye.
"tiny
taeniasis"
Hymenolepiasis
"Dwarf rats must
hide from men!"
I am not a starfish!
I am a high-to-do
ECHINOCOCCUS!
What's
happenin'
starfish?
cyst
cyst

Intestinal Nematodes: Roundworms

NOTES

⇒ Nema→Name
⇒ Tode→Toad

Hookworm

- *Necator americanus*⇒neck
- filariform larvae penetrate skin→undergo lung migration→and end up in the small intestine→eggs passed in feces
- severity of disease depends on density of worms and the patient's ability to overcome large blood loss resulting in hemorrhagic anemia from Fe^{2+} loss
- 3 signs: dermatitis, pneumonitis, hemorrhagic anemia
- treat with albendazole

Strongyloidiasis

⇒ strong arm
⇒ thread→intestinal **thread**worm

- infection due to penetration of skin by filariform larvae, then larvae are passed in feces
- larvae migrate through lungs before settling in small intestine
- external and internal autoinfection common
- no male is needed for reproduction (♀) (parthenogenetic females)
- 3 signs: dermatitis, pneumonitis, duodenitis
- treat with albendazole or ivermectin

Ascariasis

⇒ **nascar**

- eggs, found in soil, are infective
- larvae migrate through lungs and settle in small intestine
- humans only reservoir
- treat with albendazole
- complications include blocked lumen

Trichuriasis (Whipworm)

⇒ treacherous whipworm

- eggs, found in soil, are infective after maturation
- humans only host
- adult worms stay in large intestine
- children may experience rectal prolapse
- no larval lung migration
- treat with albendazole

Enterobiasis (Pinworms)

⇒ terrorist pinworm

- infective eggs deposited by female in perianal area (naked man's butt) at night
- humans only host, most often children
- autoinfection occurs through eggs but retroinfection is caused by larval form
- lower intestinal tract involved with infection
- symptoms in children include perianal itching
- dwell only in lumen as commensals
- adults are asymptomatic
- treat with albendazole

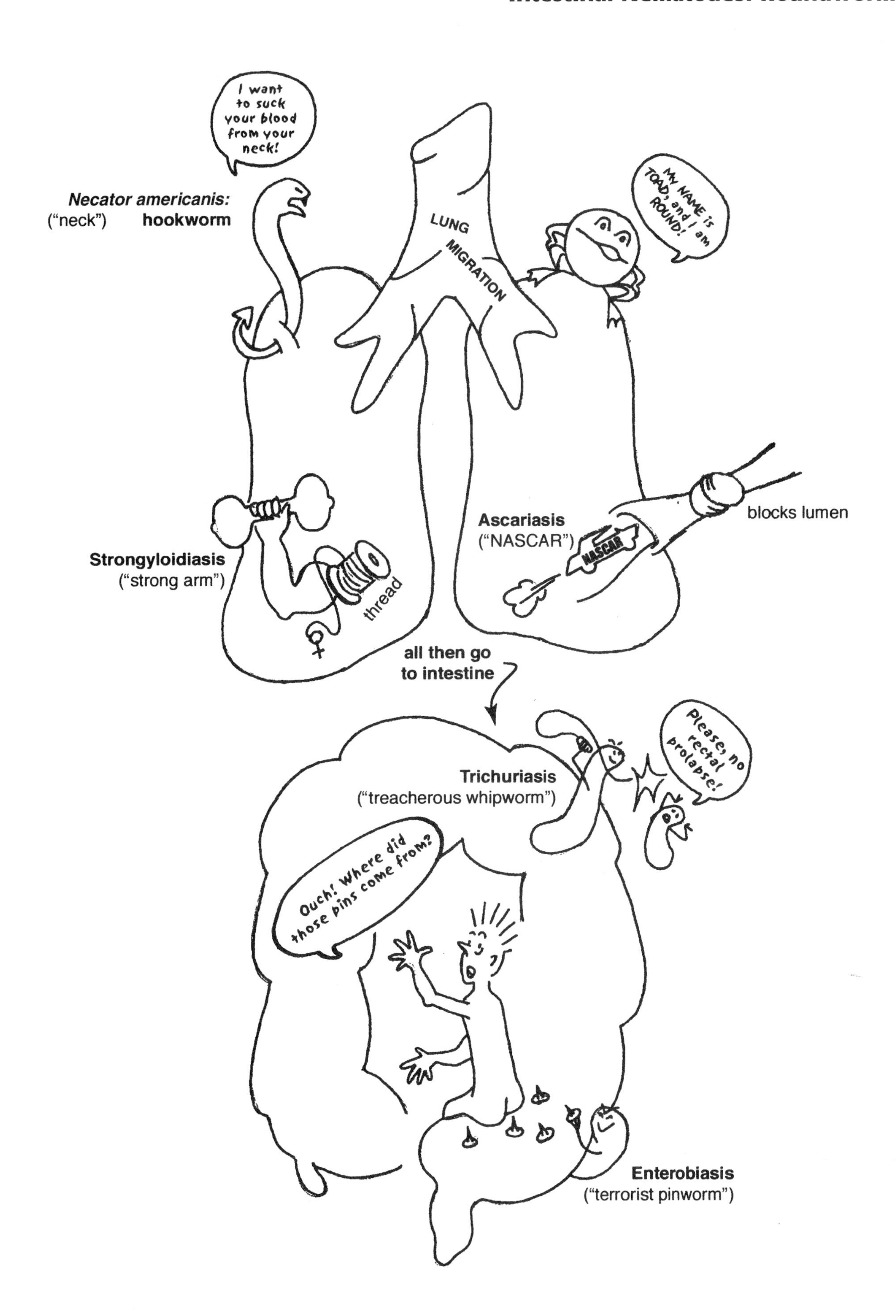
I want to suck your blood from your neck!
Necator americanis: ("neck") hookworm
LUNG MIGRATION
MY NAME is TOAD, and I am ROUND!
Strongyloidiasis ("strong arm")
thread
Ascariasis ("NASCAR")
NASCAR
blocks lumen
all then go to intestine
Trichuriasis ("treacherous whipworm")
Please, no rectal prolapse!
Ouch! Where did those pins come from?
Enterobiasis ("terrorist pinworm")

NOTES

ROUNDWORMS

⇒ tissue→tissue nematodes
⇒ name toad→nematode
⇒ round→roundworm

Visceral Larval Migrans

- eggs are ingested from fecally contaminated soil
- cannot mature in humans
- dog and cat ascarids
- viscera: liver, lung, eye
- treat with corticosteroid + thiabendazole

Cutaneous Larval Migrans

- filariform larvae of dog and cat hookworms are infectious
- penetrate skin from fecal infested soil
- treat with albendazole or local freezing

Trichinosis

⇒ tricky nose

- caused by *Trichinella spiralis*
- infection caused by ingestion of undercooked pork
- whole life cycle in one host
- adults reside in small intestine (intestinal nematode), whereas larvae reside in striated muscle (where they encyst within a fibrous capsule)
- 3 signs:
  1) duodenitis→intestinal phase with diarrhea
  2) vasculitis→migrating phase through blood vessels
  3) myositis→encysting phase
- treat with albendazole or mebendazole with corticosteroid

Dracunculiasis (Guinea Worm)

⇒ Dracula
⇒ guinea pig

- infection caused by ingesting infected cope**pod**s in fresh **water**
  ⇒ "pod in water"
  ⇒ copepods a.k.a. crustaceans
- female lives in subcutaneous tissue (will notice head of worm in skin ulcer)
- treatment with mebendazole or extraction of worm by winding upon a stick

Lymphatic Filariasis

- mosquito transmits infective larvae during bite
- scrotal lymphatics preferred by adult nematodes
- elephantiasis results after repeated inflammatory episodes and connective tissue hyperplasia

Diethylcarbamazine

- used to treat elephantiasis and loiasis

Loiasis (African Eye Worm)

- infective larvae transmitted by mango (deer) fly
- no nodule, therefore, migrating

Onchocerciasis (River Blindness)

- transmitted by black fly
- humans only reservoir
- hypersensitivity to microfilariae in skin, lymphatics, and eye causes river blindness

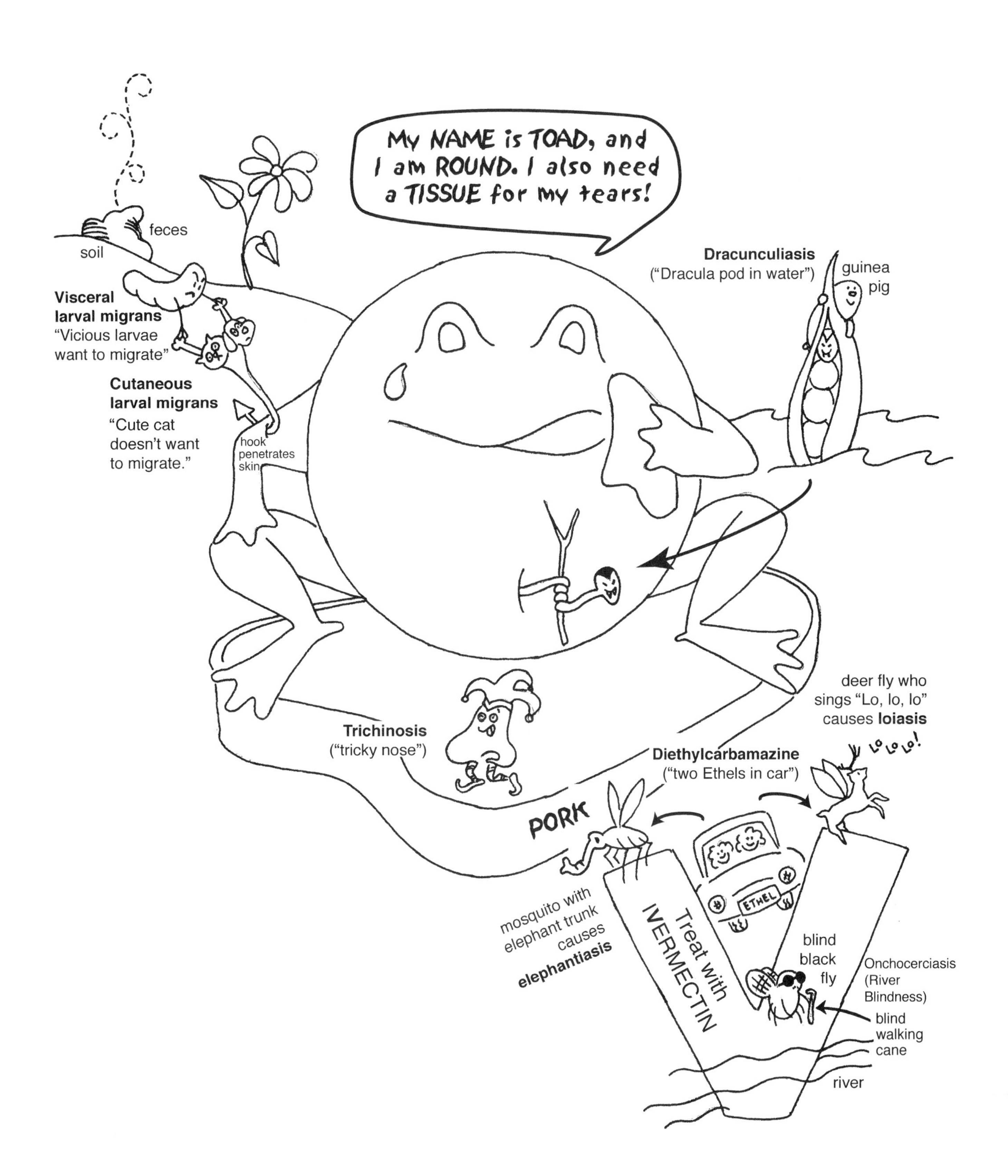
My NAME is TOAD, and I am ROUND. I also need a TISSUE for my tears!
feces
soil
Visceral larval migrans
"Vicious larvae want to migrate"
Cutaneous larval migrans
"Cute cat doesn't want to migrate."
hook penetrates skin
Dracunculiasis
("Dracula pod in water")
guinea pig
Trichinosis
("tricky nose")
PORK
deer fly who sings "Lo, lo, lo" causes loiasis
Lo Lo Lo!
Diethylcarbamazine
("two Ethels in car")
ETHEL
mosquito with elephant trunk causes elephantiasis
Treat with IVERMECTIN
blind black fly
Onchocerciasis (River Blindness)
blind walking cane
river

II.
BACTERIOLOGY

NOTES

STAPHYLOCOCCI

⇒ staff made of cocci

- gram-positive
- grow in clusters/short chains (4 or less)
- 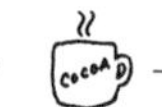 → coagulase producing
- cannot be distinguished from other gram-positive on morphological grounds alone
- exudates should always be cultured on blood agar
- the properties that correlate best with pathogenicity are DNAse and coagulase
- cause:
  - inflammatory disease:
    organ abscesses, pneumonia,
    skin infections
  - disease mediated by toxins:
    rapid-onset food poisoning (ingestion of preformed enterotoxins), TSS,
    scalded-skin syndrome

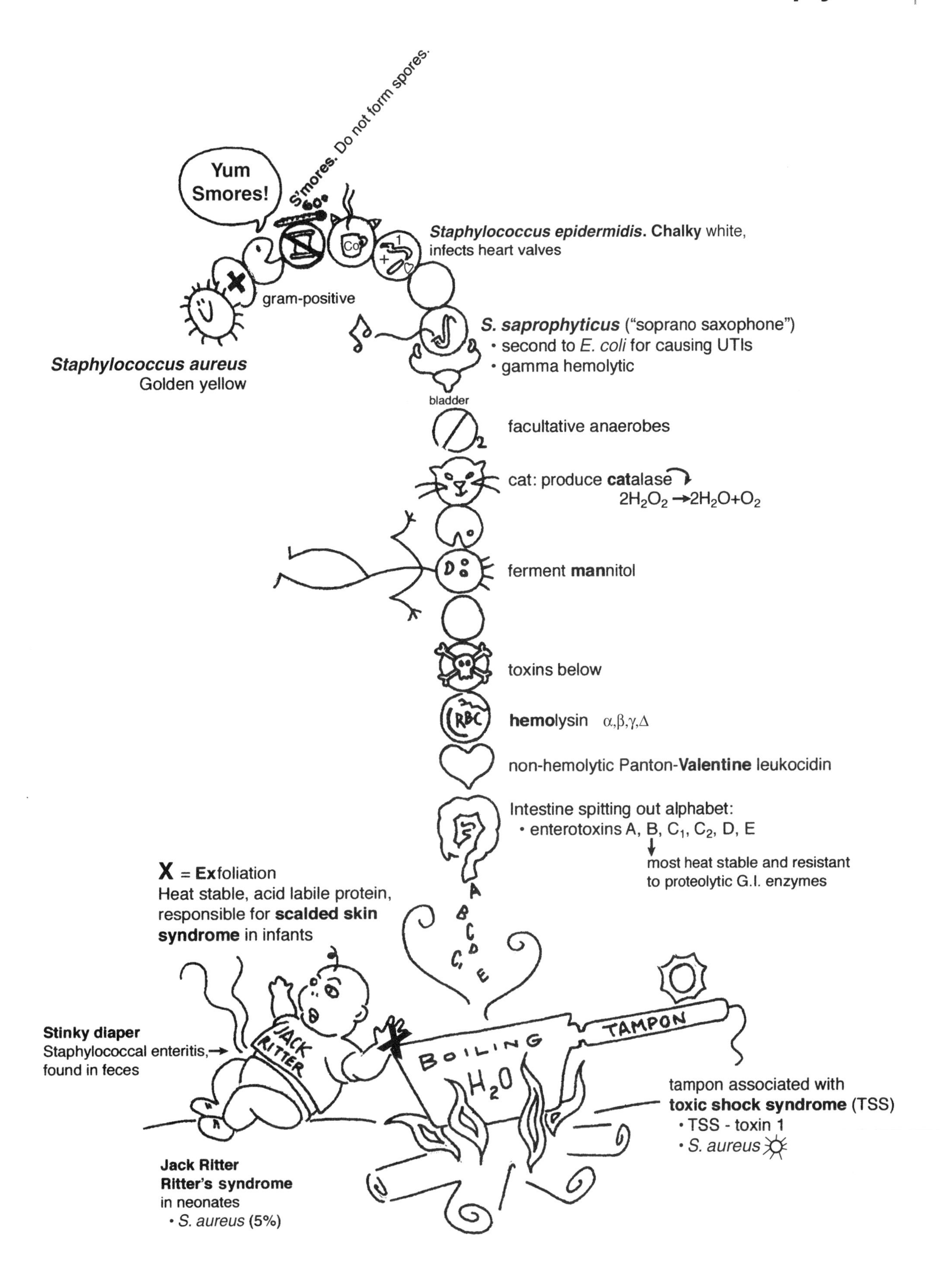
Yum Smores!
S'mores. Do not form spores.
60°
Co
Staphylococcus epidermidis. Chalky white, infects heart valves
gram-positive
Staphylococcus aureus
Golden yellow
S. saprophyticus ("soprano saxophone")
• second to E. coli for causing UTIs
• gamma hemolytic
bladder
facultative anaerobes
cat: produce catalase
$2H_2O_2 \rightarrow 2H_2O + O_2$
ferment mannitol
toxins below
RBC
hemolysin α,β,γ,Δ
non-hemolytic Panton-Valentine leukocidin
Intestine spitting out alphabet:
• enterotoxins A, B, C_1, C_2, D, E
most heat stable and resistant to proteolytic G.I. enzymes
X = Exfoliation
Heat stable, acid labile protein, responsible for scalded skin syndrome in infants
A
B
C
D
C,
E
Stinky diaper
Staphylococcal enteritis, found in feces
JACK RITTER
BOILING
H_2O
TAMPON
tampon associated with
toxic shock syndrome (TSS)
• TSS - toxin 1
• S. aureus
Jack Ritter
Ritter's syndrome
in neonates
• S. aureus (5%)

NOTES

STREPTOCOCCUS

⇒ causes strep throat
α-hemolytic—turn green
β-hemolytic—clear zone
γ—no reaction
gram-positive

α-HEMOLYTIC

Streptococcus viridans

⇒ virility dance steps
- α-hemolytic
- *S. mutans* causes dental caries
  ⇒ mutates teeth
- leading cause of subacute bacterial endocarditis
  ⇒ dancing to heart
  ⇒ slow-forming

Streptococcus pneumoniae

⇒ lungs
alpha-hemolytic→α-shape in
diplococci- 2α's make
lancet-shaped→ ancet
lung→quellung reaction
- normally gram-positive up to and including exponential phase of growth, but usually become gram-negative after that; bile salts stimulate change by autolysis
- smooth capsule→more virulent
  ⇒ smooth cap
- presence of these bacteria is only significant in presence of white blood cells
- differentiate from *S. viridans* by bile solubility and optochin sensitivity
- use penicillin to treat infection
- associated with sepsis in sickle cell anemia, splenectomy, and rusty sputum

β-HEMOLYTIC

Group A: *Streptococcus pyogenes*

⇒ pie on jeans
- **Suppurative Disease**
  ⇒ streptococcal pharyngitis, scarlet fever
- Non-suppurative sequelae
  ⇒ acute glomerulonephritis, rheumatic fever
- **Treatment is penicillin**
  ⇒ penny→penicillin

M→M antibodies are protective
5 Toxins:
"Hiya, Ron!"→capsular hyaluronic acid
FAT →lipoteichoic acid
⇒ mediates adherence to buccal epithelial cells
streptokinase→RBC lysis
S, O→streptolysins S and O

Group B: β-Hemolytic

⇒ *S. **aga**lactiae* ⇒ AGA!
- WAH, WAH!→baby crying
  ⇒ important cause of neonatal disease
- can cause "early disease"
  ⇒ sepsis, lung involvement, meningitis (serotype III)
- can cause "late disease"
  ⇒ occurs after a week to one month postpartum
  ⇒ associated with meningitis (serotype III)

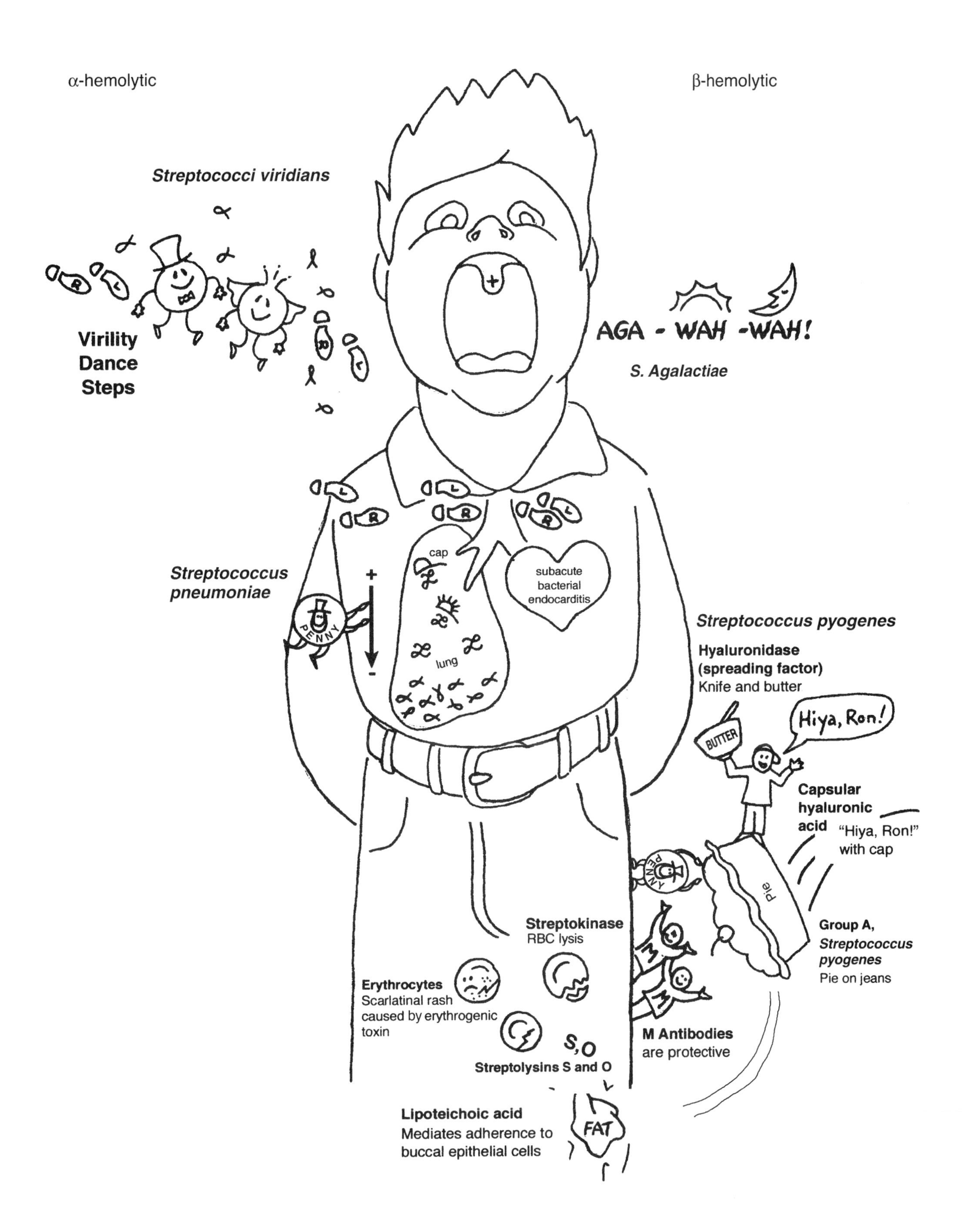
α-hemolytic
β-hemolytic
Streptococci viridians
Virility
Dance
Steps
AGA - WAH -WAH!
S. Agalactiae
Streptococcus
pneumoniae
PENNY
cap
lung
subacute
bacterial
endocarditis
Streptococcus pyogenes
Hyaluronidase
(spreading factor)
Knife and butter
BUTTER
Hiya, Ron!
Capsular
hyaluronic
acid
"Hiya, Ron!"
with cap
PENNY
Pie
Group A,
Streptococcus
pyogenes
Pie on jeans
Streptokinase
RBC lysis
Erythrocytes
Scarlatinal rash
caused by erythrogenic
toxin
S,O
Streptolysins S and O
M Antibodies
are protective
Lipoteichoic acid
Mediates adherence to
buccal epithelial cells
FAT

NOTES

Bacillus anthracis

⇒ Athens

- spore-forming⇒smore
- Medusa head appearance under hand-held lens
- treat with penicillin and tetracycline
  ⇒ penny ⇒ tetracycle
  used for treatment
- facultative anaerobe
  ⇒ O_2 or $\emptyset_2$
- causes woolsorter's disease

Corynebacterium diphtheriae

⇒ club-shaped corn growing on Dippy's head

- club-shaped on artificial media
- non-spore-forming⇒no s'mores
- beta-phage required for toxin production
  ⇒ toxin ↑ with low Fe^{2+}
- causes diphtheria in humans
- antitoxin used to treat immediately→ antibiotic therapy should never be relied on alone
- humans only reservoir
- get pseudomembrane

Bacillus cereus

⇒ serious bacillus

- insensitive to penicillin
  ⇒ knock out penny
- food poisoning (caused by spores) two syndromes
  1) 4-hr manifestation
     ⇒ vomiting
  2) >20-hr incubation⇒diarrhea
- treat with clindamycin
  ⇒ clink
  ⇒ drug of choice

Listeria monocytogenes

⇒ Hysterical Lisa

- only gram(+) that produces endotoxin
- most distinctive infection is in genital tract of gravid female with infection of neonate
- penicillin G→drug of choice
- exotoxin→Lysterolysin O
- high fatality rate for neonates (early infection causes stillbirth and late infection causes meningitis)
- motile by peritrichous flagella
- get it from ingesting dairy products and deli meats

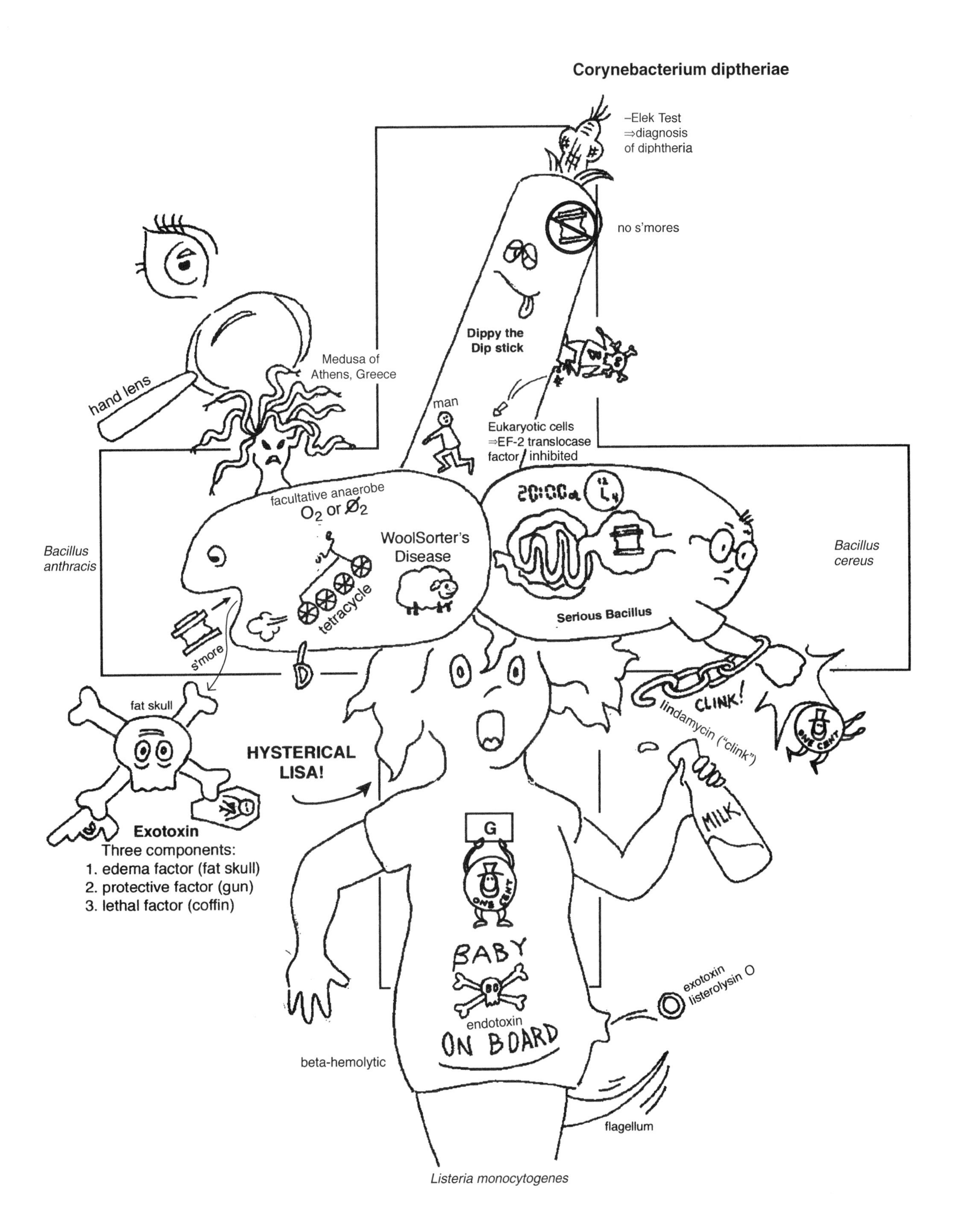
Corynebacterium diptheriae
–Elek Test
⇒diagnosis
of diphtheria
no s'mores
Dippy the
Dip stick
Medusa of
Athens, Greece
hand lens
man
Eukaryotic cells
⇒EF-2 translocase
factor / inhibited
facultative anaerobe
O2 or Ø2
WoolSorter's
Disease
tetracycle
s'more
Bacillus
anthracis
Serious Bacillus
Bacillus
cereus
CLINK!
lindamycin ("clink")
ONE CENT
MILK
fat skull
HYSTERICAL
LISA!
G
ONE CENT
BABY
endotoxin
ON BOARD
exotoxin
listerolysin O
Exotoxin
Three components:
1. edema factor (fat skull)
2. protective factor (gun)
3. lethal factor (coffin)
beta-hemolytic
flagellum
Listeria monocytogenes

NOTES

Cephalosporins (cellophane)

- from mold
  1) bactericidal
  2) parenterally/orally administered
  3) side effect→hypersensitivity
- 6-ring structure

Bacitracin→Tracy's Back

1) produced by *Bacillus subtilis*
2) inhibits peptidoglycan synthesis by preventing (Tracy kicking sugar cube) the attachment of amino sugars to cell membrane lipids ()
3) bactericidal against multiplying bacteria
   - nephrotoxic⇒kidneys in back

Cycloserine

⇒ cyclone and serene

my→kills *Mycobacterium tuberculosis*

- central nervous system toxicity
- inhibits D-alanine use in synthesis of bacterial cell wall

Beta-Lactam Antimicrobial Agents

M = monobactams
= penems
CD = carbapenems

- cause seizures

Inhibitors—Administered in Combination with Beta-Lactam Antimicrobial Agents

"Tim the inhibitor, augments u in the zoo."
Tim = Timentin
augment = Augmentin
u = Unasyn
zoo = Zosyn

Penicillin

⇒ Penny

1) interferes with synthesis of peptidoglycan
   ⇒ cap on Pepsi bottle
2) binds outer cell membrane proteins
   A) carboxypeptidases⇒carbonation
   B) transpeptidases⇒traverses
3) activate autolytic enzymes
   ⇒ crack in bottle
4) bactericidal against actively multiplying cells
   G—narrow spectrum (highly potent)
   V—narrow spectrum (low potent)
   - penicilloyl—hapten responsible for hypersensitivity
   - cause GI disturbances
   - 5-ring structure
   - tolerance:
     ⇒ low MIC (minimum inhibitory concentration)
     ⇒ high MBC (minimum bactericidal concentration)
   - use low dose to stop and high dose to kill

Vancomycin

⇒ Van

amino sugars⇒mean sugar cubes

1) inhibits transfer of amino sugars to the growing end of glycopeptide on cell wall
2) bactericidal against multiplying bacteria
3) neurotoxicity—auditory nerve damage with hearing loss
   ⇒ WHAT?
   - narrow spectrum

β→Beta Lactamase—resides in periplasmic space of gram-negative bacteria; degrades penicillins

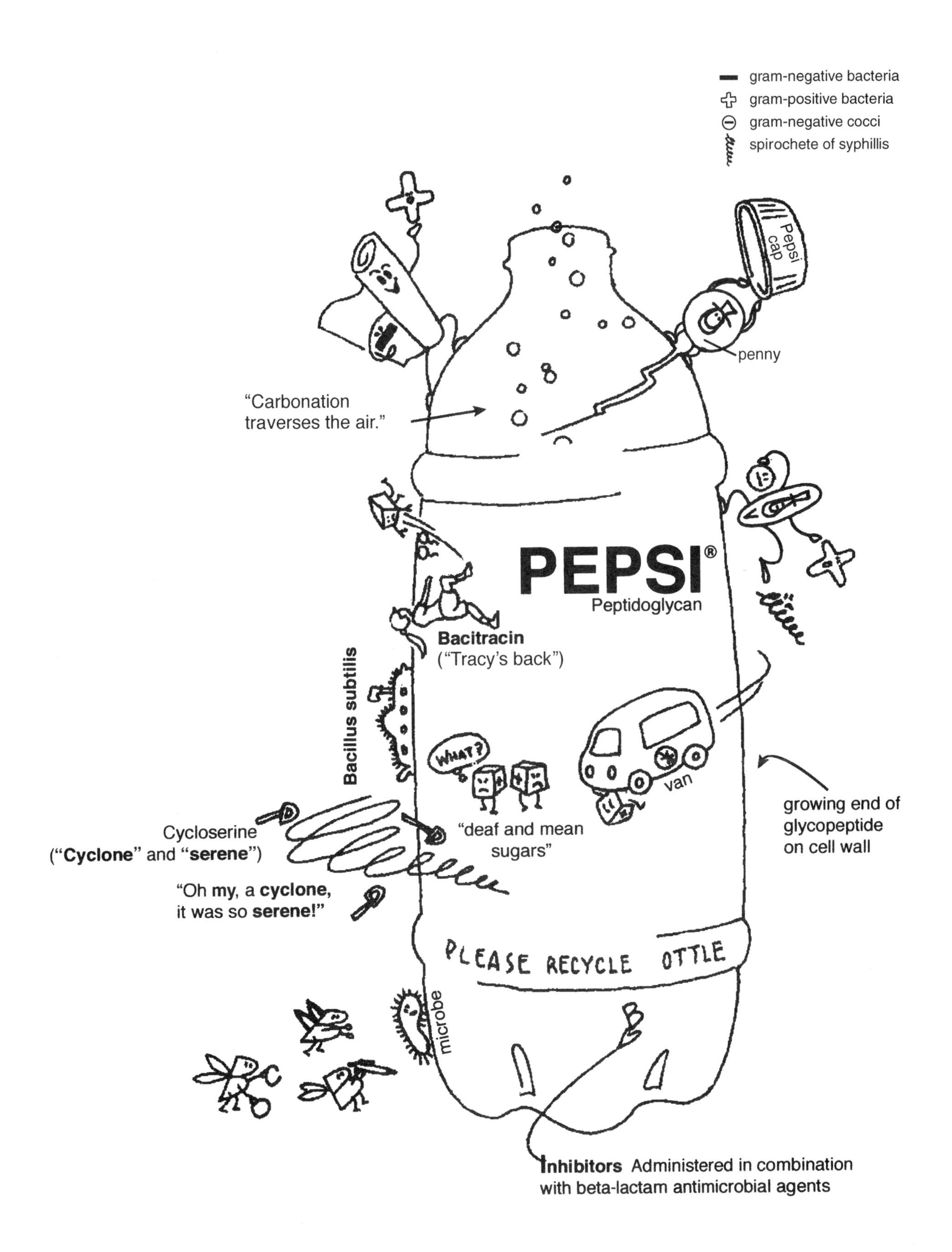
gram-negative bacteria
gram-positive bacteria
gram-negative cocci
spirochete of syphillis
Pepsi cap
penny
"Carbonation traverses the air."
PEPSI®
Peptidoglycan
Bacitracin
("Tracy's back")
Bacillus subtilis
WHAT?
van
"deaf and mean sugars"
growing end of glycopeptide on cell wall
Cycloserine
("**Cyclone**" and "**serene**")
"Oh **my**, a **cyclone**, it was so **serene!**"
PLEASE RECYCLE OTTLE
microbe
Inhibitors Administered in combination with beta-lactam antimicrobial agents

NOTES

Rifamycin

⇒ (RIF)
- inhibits bacterial DNA-dependent RNA polymerase
- broad spectrum
  ⇒ broad tombstone
- primarily used against *Mycobacterium tuberculosis*
  ⇒ TB on tombstone

Quinolone (derivative of nalidixic acid)

⇒ (**Quint**alope **alone**)⇒5 horns
- inhibits bacterial DNA gyrase
- broad spectrum (many horns)
- **enox**acin, **norflox**acin, **cip**rofloxacin
  ⇒ enox ⇒ north flock ⇒ skip
- "Enox skipped to north to join ox flock"

Metronidazole

⇒ (**Metro** runs **ni**ght and **da**y!)
- MOA→4 steps
  1) passive diffusion of metronidazole into target cell
  2) metronidazole activated by reduction
  3) toxic intermediates
     ⇒ single and double strands break in DNA
  4) release of inactive end products
- narrow spectrum
  ⇒ anaerobic bacteria and anaerobic protozoa
  (*Trichomonas vaginalis*)
  ⇒ "Tricky Mona"

Side effects:
- mutagenic and carcinogenic in animals
- peripheral neuropathy
- disulfiram-like reaction with alcohol

Nalidixic Acid

⇒ (**Nal**'s—**Dixi**e)
- inhibits DNA gyrase
- narrow spectrum
  ⇒ gram-negative bacilli⇒slit ▭ in door
- used primarily in UTIs
  ⇒ outhouse means UTIs

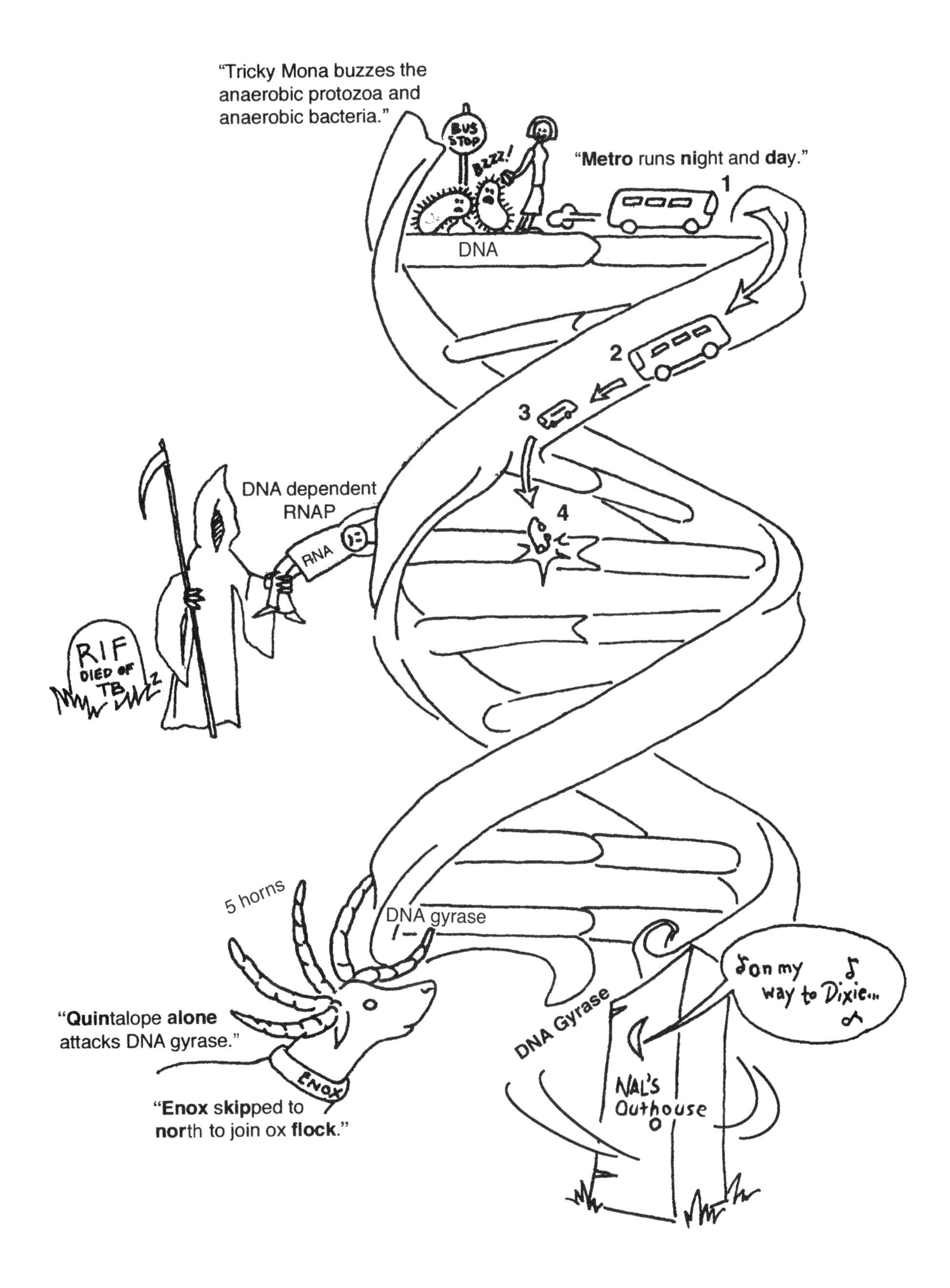
"Tricky Mona buzzes the anaerobic protozoa and anaerobic bacteria."
BUS STOP
BZZZ!
"Metro runs night and day."
1
DNA
2
3
4
DNA dependent RNAP
RNA
RIF DIED OF TB
5 horns
DNA gyrase
"Quintalope alone attacks DNA gyrase."
ENOX
"Enox skipped to north to join ox flock."
DNA Gyrase
On my way to Dixie...
NAL'S Outhouse

Antimicrobial Agents Inhibiting Folic Acid Synthesis

NOTES

- All bacterostatic⇒Foal licking acid

Sulfonamides

- ⇒ (SULFUR ON, AM I!)
- broad spectrum
  - ⇒ arms open wide
- used in UTIs, GI, and as topical
- structural analogs of *p*-aminobenzoic acid (PABA)
  - ⇒ (magician says "PABA CADABRA")
- inhibits tetrahydropteric acid synthetase
  - ⇒ 4 bubbles
- causes: anemia, thrombocytopenia, leukopenia, skin rashes

Trimethoprim

- ⇒ (**TRY MET.** IT'S **PRIME.**)
- co-trimoxazole (dog sitting on **cot**'s **rim**)
  - ⇒ mixture of trimethoprim + sulfamethoxazole→inhibits both steps of synthesis
  - ⇒ treatment of UTI, traveller's diarrhea
- competitive inhibitor of reductase dihydrofolate⇒"two water foals"

Sulfones

- ⇒ (cell phone)
- major agent is diaminodiphenylsulfone (DDS)⇒(two diamonds)
- narrow spectrum
- used in leprosy⇒(leopard)

mechanism of action of sulfonamides and trimethoprim on metabolic pathway of bacterial folic acid synthesis:

PABA
↓ ✗ SULFONAMIDES (tetrahydropteroic acid synthetase)
DIHYDROFOLIC ACID
↓ ✗ TRIMETHOPRIM (dihydrofolate reductase)
TETRAHYDROFOLIC ACID
↓
purines

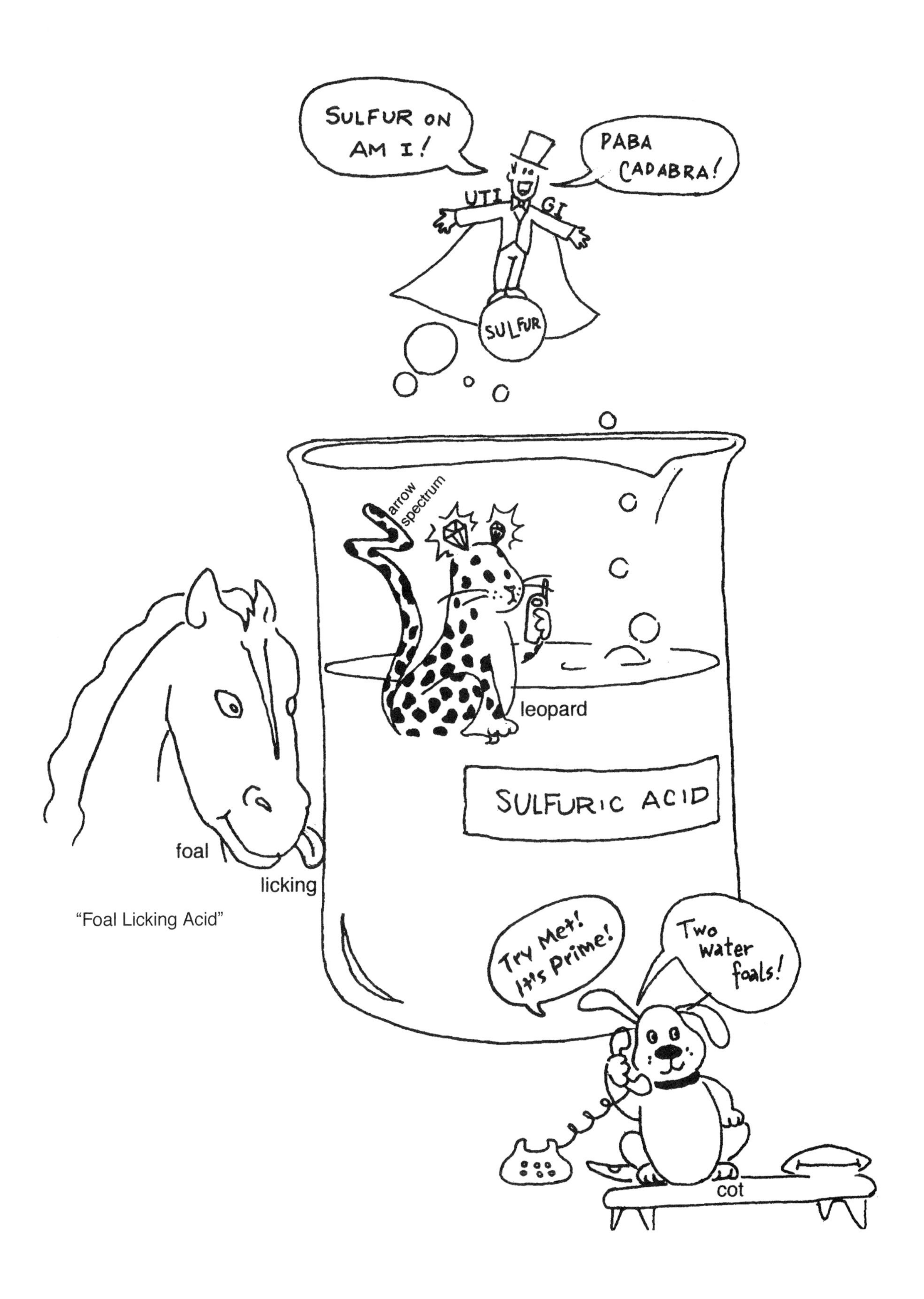
SULFUR ON AM I!
PABA CADABRA!
UTI
GI
SULFUR
arrow spectrum
leopard
SULFURIC ACID
foal
licking
"Foal Licking Acid"
Try Met! It's Prime!
Two water foals!
cot

Agents Inhibiting Protein Synthesis

NOTES

Aminoglycosides⇒"A Mean Geico Insurance Agent"

"Gentleman, Toby, and Stripper Ami sped to Kansas in a Neon."—insured by Geico
gentleman—gentamicin produced by *Micromonospora*; all others by Streptomyces; treat gram positive

- irreversibly bound to 30S () subunit
- used to treat gram negative ()

Toby = tobramycin
stripper = streptomycin
ami = amikacin
sped = spectinomycin
Kansas = kanamycin
Neon = neomycin
Side effects:
nephrotoxicity and ototoxicity
⇒ . . . WHAT?

Chloramphenicol

⇒ (colored fin)

- broad spectrum
  ⇒ broad range of colors
- reversibly binds 50S
- causes reversible bone marrow depression⇒bone
- causes (rarely) aplastic anemia and gray baby syndrome (premature infants lacking liver UDP-glucuronyl transferase)

Tetracyclines

C = chlortetracycline⇒Clorox bottle
D = doxycycline⇒DO_2x
O = oxytetracycline⇒O_2
M = minocycline⇒O_2→treatment for acne

- broad spectrum
- causes tooth discoloration⇒black tooth
- requires energy to enter cell (ATP)
  ⇒ requires energy to ride cycle
- if resistant to one tetracycline, resistant to all
- do not take with antacids because divalent cations will inhibit gut absorption of it.

Quinupristin/dalfopristin

⇒ (quints prison)
⇒ (dallas prison)

- active against gram-positive ()
- used in vancomycin-resistant *Enterococcus faecium* (VREF)
  ⇒ van
  and nosocomial diarrhea
  ⇒ nose with stuff running out
- hepatotoxicity side effect

Lincosamides

- lincomycin⇒links
- clindamycin
  ⇒ (clinks)
- same action as erythromycin primarily against anaerobic bacteria

Macrolides

⇒ (Big Mac slides)

- erythromycin⇒ERY!
- moderately broad spectrum
- binds 50S unit

"Solid Z-line"

⇒ (linezolid)

- inhibits on ribosomal level
- used in VREF and methicillin-resistant *Staphylococcus aureus*
- when combined with pseudoephedrine or phenylpropanolamine can cause increase in blood pressure

gram-negative
gram-positive
30S (Laurie is sad she is 30)
⇒ tRNA binds
50S (half of $1)
⇒ linking of growing peptide chain
(handcuffs) irreversibly bound
reversibly bound

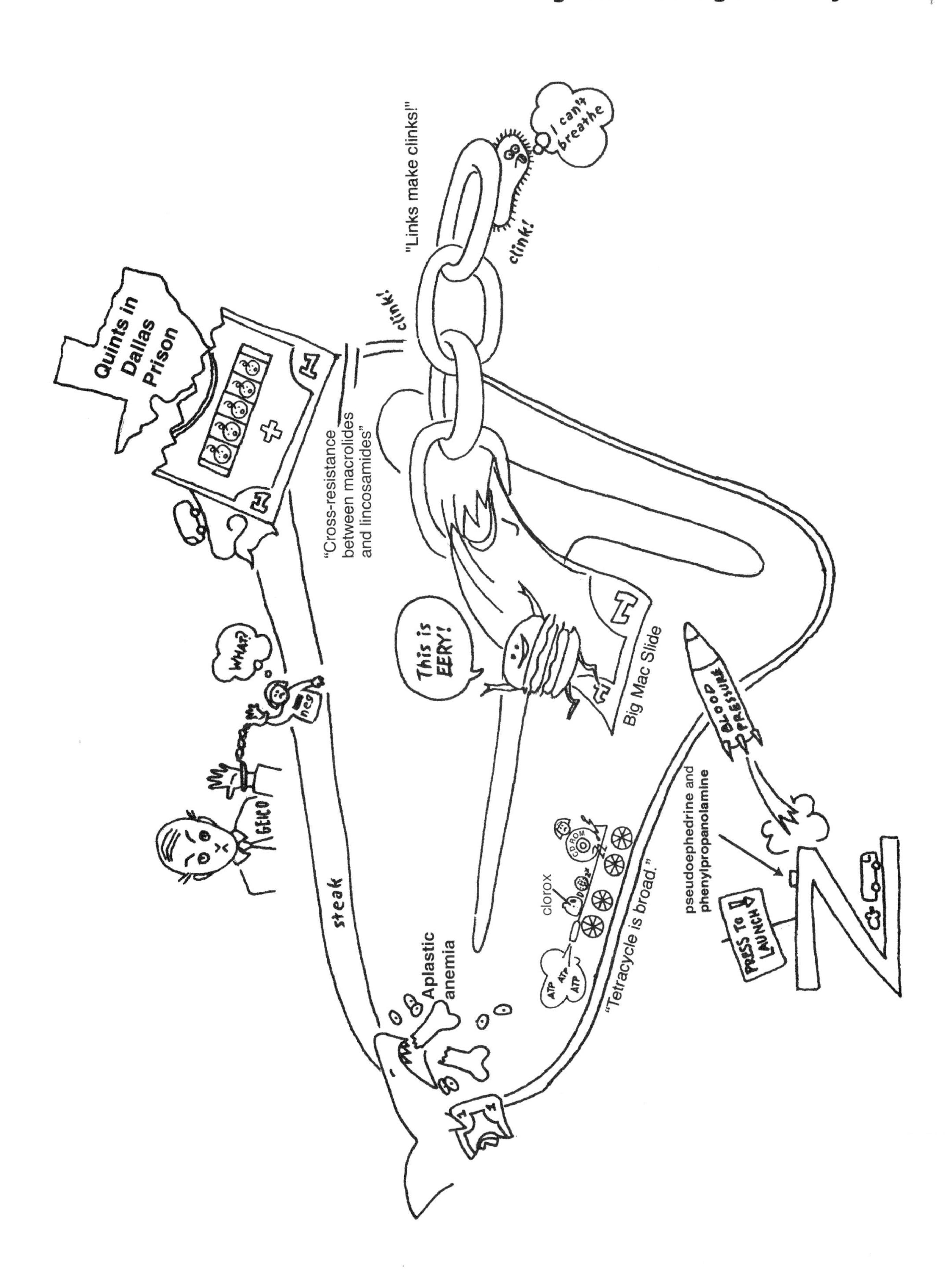
Quints in Dallas Prison
"Cross-resistance between macrolides and lincosamides"
clink!
"Links make clinks!"
clink!
I can't breathe
WHAT?
GEICO
neg
This is EERY!
Big Mac Slide
BLOOD PRESSURE
pseudoephedrine and phenylpropanolamine
PRESS TO LAUNCH
steak
Aplastic anemia
clorox
ATP
ATP
ATP
CD ROM
"Tetracycle is broad."

NOTES

POLYMYXIN

Poly A—toxic
Poly B
Poly C—toxic
Poly D—toxic
Poly E—same as colistin
⇒ (cloned)

- functions as a cationic detergent which disrupts osmotic integrity of cell membrane
- narrow spectrum of gram-negative bacilli
  - ⇒ negative
- topical ointments
  - ⇒ usually in combination with neomycin (neon) or bacitracin (Tracy's back)
- neurotoxic, nephrotoxic

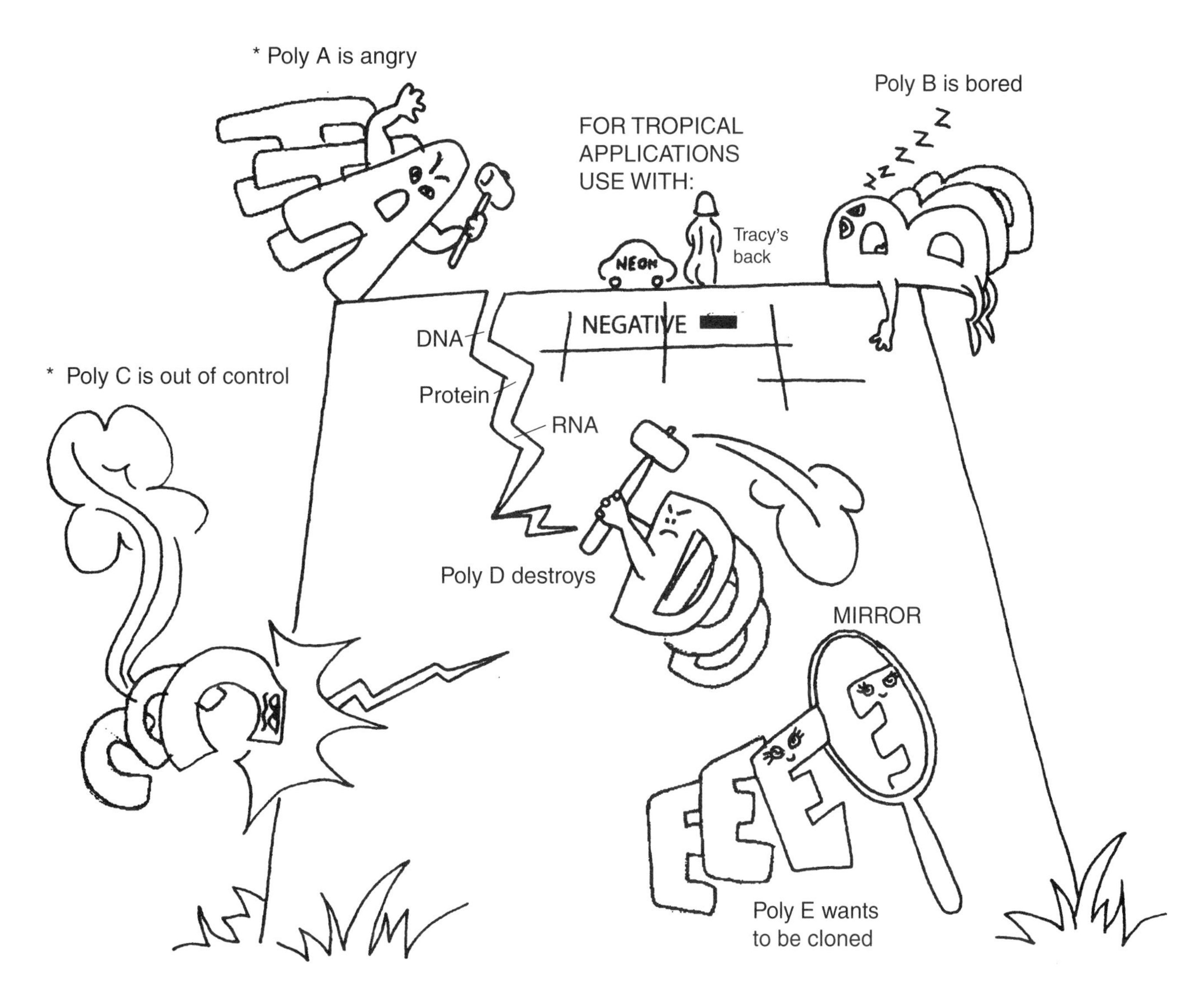

* Toxic ones are destroying wall

NOTES

ISONIAZID

- ⇒ (I saw a night alien)
- analog of B-6
  - ⇒ (6 bees)
- a.k.a. pyridoxine
  - ⇒ (Pirate with dots)
- treatment for *Mycobacterium* TB
  - ⇒ (coughing bees)
  - ⇒ (TB on pants)

NITROFURANS

- ⇒ nitro carrying furry ants
- used for UTIs
  - ⇒ (outhouse)
- broad spectrum

ETHAMBUTOL

- ⇒ ET, ham, buttercup
- treatment for *Mycobacterium* TB
- rare side effects related to eyes
  - ⇒ (ET's **eyes** are big)

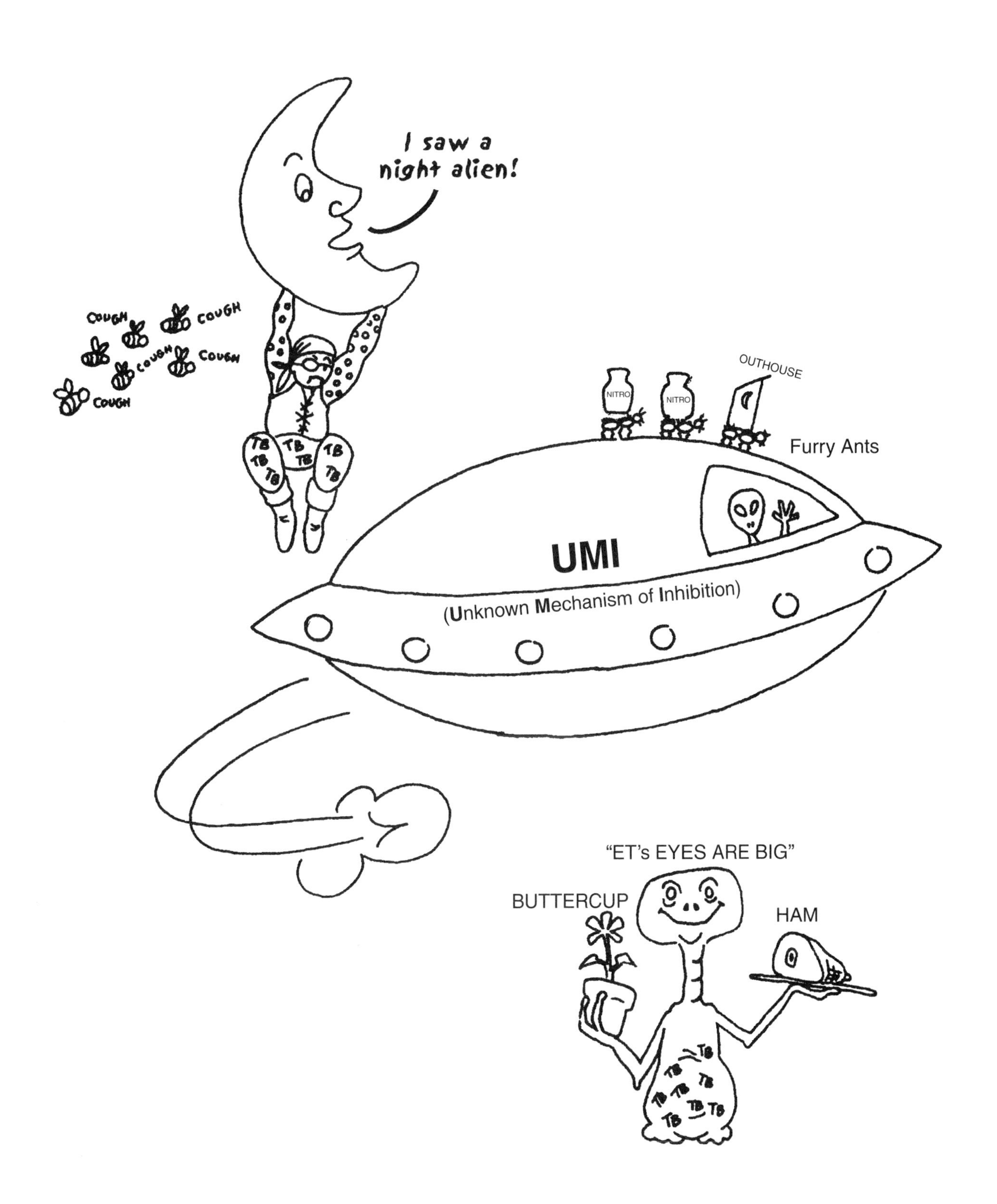
I saw a night alien!
COUGH
COUGH
COUGH
COUGH
COUGH
TB
NITRO
NITRO
OUTHOUSE
Furry Ants
UMI
(Unknown Mechanism of Inhibition)
"ET's EYES ARE BIG"
BUTTERCUP
HAM

NOTES

RODS OF INDIGENOUS FLORA

⇒ antigens as flowers, stems, and leaves and large flower in middle of colon

ANTIGENICITY

O-antigen

- part of outer membrane of cell wall
- lipopolysaccharide in composition
- O-specific chains containing repeating units of hexoses extend out from the core
- smooth (S) to rough (R) dissociation occurs in mutants that fail to synthesize part or all the O-specific chains resulting in loss of O-antigenicity

K-antigen

- capsular antigen covering O-antigen (polysaccharide)

H-antigen

- associated with flagella
- protein in composition

Endotoxin

- lipid A→toxic fraction ( )
- attached to the core of O-antigen complex
- causes-pyrogenicity (HOT!)

Types of Infections produced outside the intestine by enteric bacteria

—abscesses
headache—meningitis
cough/lungs—pneumonia
—septicemia
—wound infections
—endocarditis
toilet—UTIs

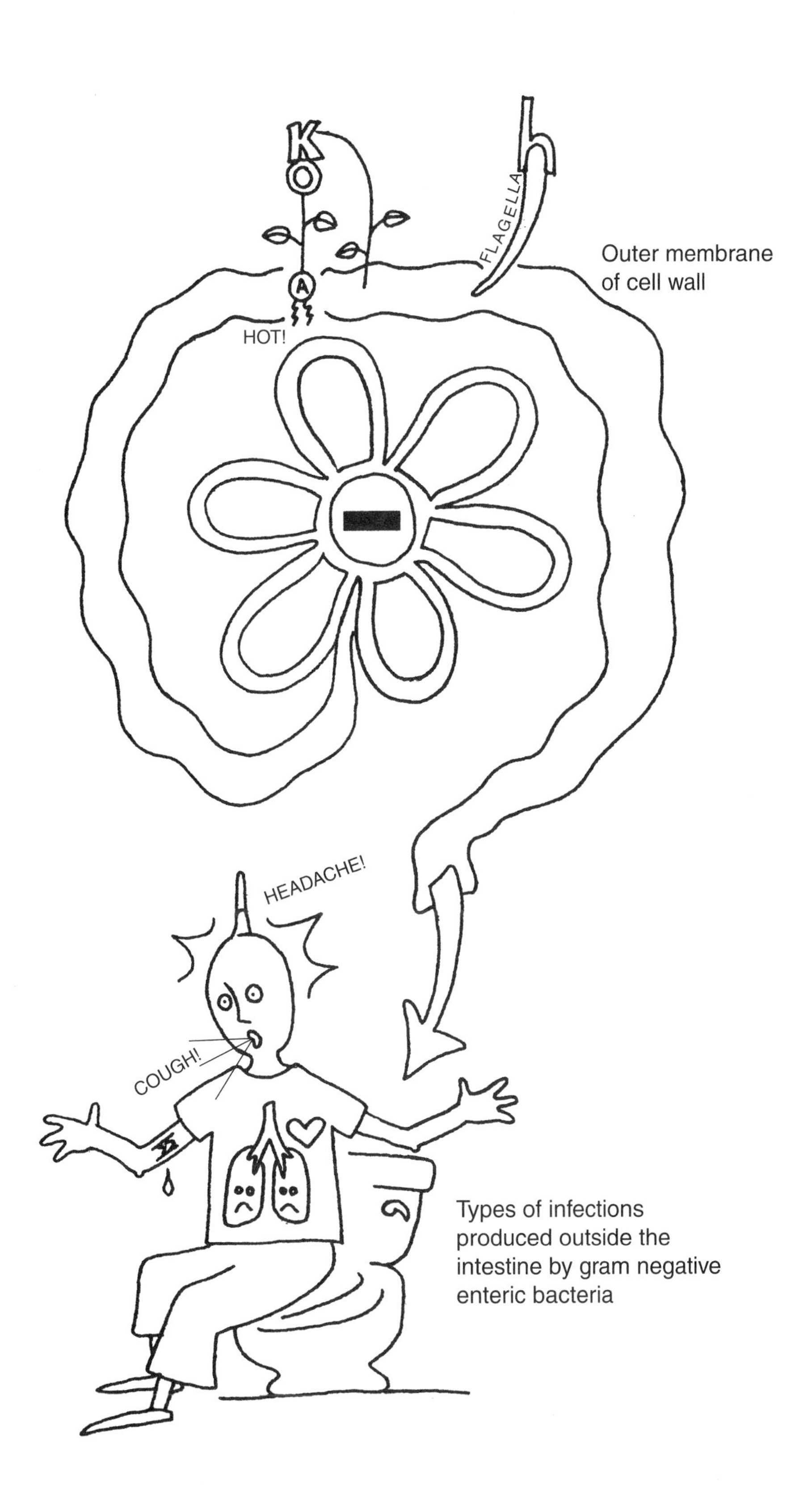
K
O
A
HOT!
FLAGELLA
Outer membrane
of cell wall
HEADACHE!
COUGH!
Types of infections
produced outside the
intestine by gram negative
enteric bacteria

NOTES

PRINCIPAL ENTEROTOXIN PRODUCERS EXCEPT *E. COLI* PATHOGENIC

Vibrio cholerae

⇒ (vibrating comma)
⇒ motile

- comma-shaped
- produces acid (upset stomach) but **no** gas from carbohydrates
- capable of growing at very high PHs (BASIC)
- biotypes
  i. classical
  ii. El Tor (hemolytic)
  ⇒ classic cholera produced by strains which belong to serogroup 0:1
  ⇒ serotypes of serogroup 0:1
    i. O-antigens A, B (ogawa)
    ii. O-antigens A, C (Inaba)
- no animal reservoirs
- infected humans transmit organism through feces
- water-borne transmission
- new strain—serogroup 0:139 (Bengal cholerae)
  ⇒ indistinguishable systems from *V. cholerae* 0:1
  ⇒ fears may initiate new pandemic
  ⇒ frequent resistance to antimicrobials
- attachment of organism at small intestine brush border
- exotoxin (choleragen)
  A_1-toxicity⇒"A"
  A_2-facilitates entry
  B region (choleragenoid) consists of 5 peptide chains
  ⇒ responsible for binding of toxin to GM1 by ADP ribosylation of G-protein ganglioside receptor of epithelial cell membrane
- enterotoxin MOA
  1) increased adenylate cyclase activity
  2) hypersecretion Cl^- and HCO_3^-
  3) prevention of Na^+ and Cl^- absorption into cells
  4) accompanying secretion of fluid into lumen
- rice water stools

Enteropathogenic *E. coli*

⇒ cold *E. coli*
⇒ Patty→Pathogenic

- predilection for bottle fed infants
- diarrhea in developing countries
- does not produce enterotoxin

Enterotoxigenic *E. coli*

- attach to small intestine epithelial cells by pili with CFA (**colon**ization factor)
  heat LT— heat labile like cholera toxin
  heat ST (stable)—↑ guanylate cyclase activity
- toxin controlled by plasmid
- causes watery diarrhea

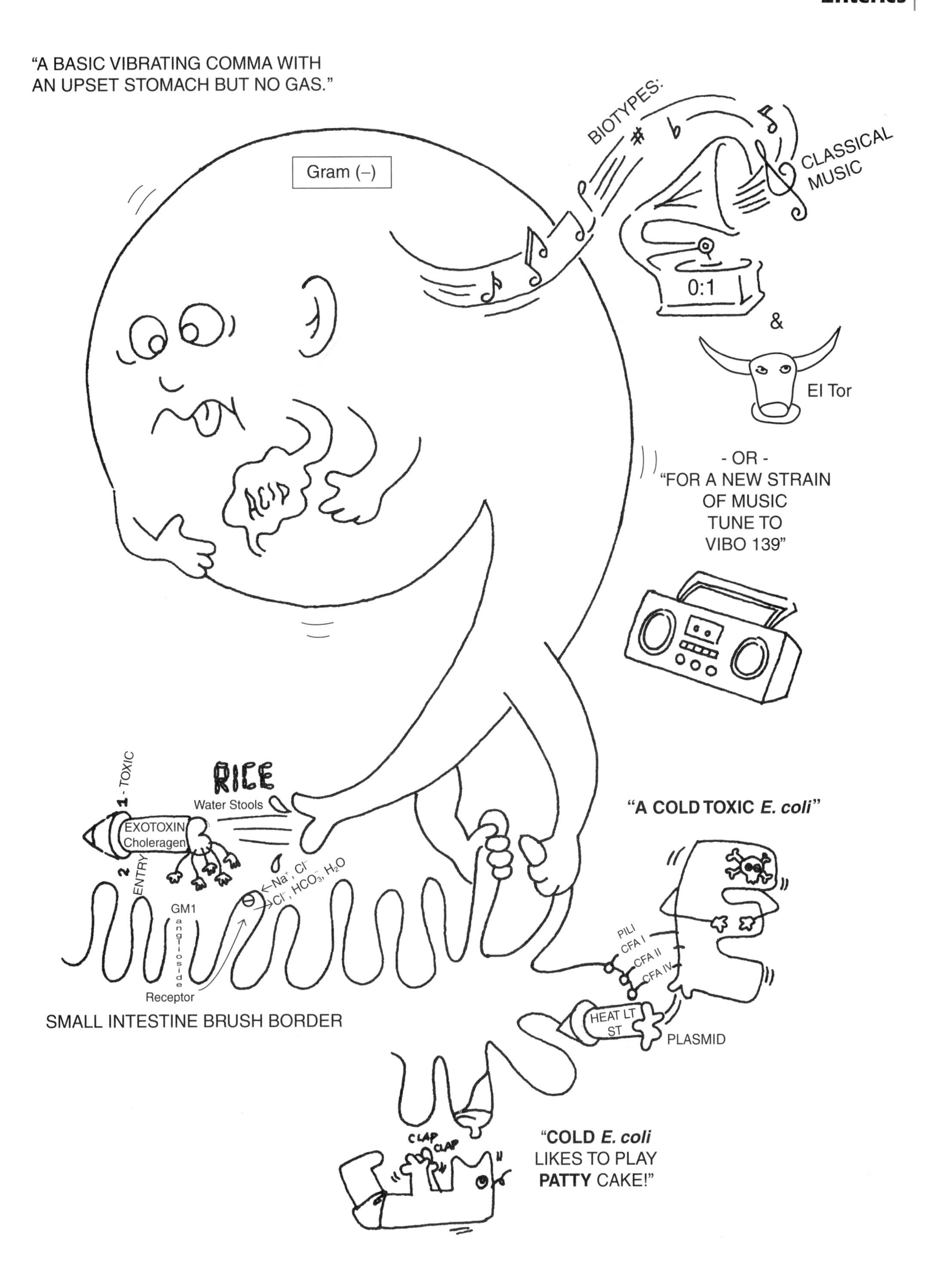
"A BASIC VIBRATING COMMA WITH
AN UPSET STOMACH BUT NO GAS."
Gram (–)
BIOTYPES:
CLASSICAL
MUSIC
0:1
&
El Tor
ACID
- OR -
"FOR A NEW STRAIN
OF MUSIC
TUNE TO
VIBO 139"
1 - TOXIC
RICE
Water Stools
EXOTOXIN
Choleragen
2 ENTRY
←Na⁺, Cl⁻
→Cl⁻, HCO₃⁻, H₂O
GM1
angliosside
Receptor
SMALL INTESTINE BRUSH BORDER
"A COLD TOXIC E. coli"
PILI
CFA I
CFA II
CFA IV
HEAT LT
ST
PLASMID
CLAP
CLAP
"COLD E. coli
LIKES TO PLAY
PATTY CAKE!"

NOTES

BACTERIA OF GREATEST MEDICAL IMPORTANCE

Coliform Organisms

⇒ cauliflower

cold *E. coli*—*Escherichia coli*
Kleb—*Klebsiella* species
"Into racing"—*Enterobacter* species
site and row—*Citrobacter* species
Sierra—*Serratia* species

E. coli

⇒ cold *E. coli*

- inhabits intestinal tract (colon) exclusively

—ferments carbohydrates
+ lactose→acid and gas
⇒ upset stomach

—K_1 antigen responsible for neonatal meningitis

- antigenically heterogeneous O, K, H antigens
- some *E. coli* strains are intestinal pathogens

Proteus Species

- "A **Morgan-UREA** accountant with an upset stomach and gas counted **protein** beans in **Providencce**, RI. He also complained of basic urine and calculi."

Protein—*Proteus*
Morgan—*Morganella*
Providence—*Providencia*

- ferment carbohydrates but not lactose
- important species
  Proteus mirabilis
  Proteus vulgaris
  Morganella morganii
  Providencia rettgeri
- these organisms hydrolyze urea to produce CO_2 and ammonia→resulting in ↑PH of urine causing precipitation of CA^{2+} and Mg phosphates and formation of calculi

Enterobacteria

⇒ "into racing bacteria"

Klebsiella
⇒ Kleb-siesta

- enterobacteria are motile
  ⇒ car is motile
- *Klebsiella* are non-motile
  ⇒ isn't going anywhere after being hit by car
- ferment carbohydrates and lactose producing acid (**upset stom**ach) and **gas**

lung—*Klebsiella pneumoniae,* which is heavily encapsulated, produces acute pneumonia in debilitated individuals

Pseudomonas Aeruginosa

- ubiquitous in nature—soil, water, intestinal tract—and hospital equipment
- aerobes do not ferment carbohydrates
- produces blue-green H_2O-soluble pigments
- virulence factors—endotoxin, slime layer, leukocidin, enzymes, exotoxin A
- Opportunistic infections
  ⇒ "Many opportunities if you own a pseudo rug."
- exotoxin A inactivates EF-2 (elongation factor 2)
  ⇒ required for translocation of polypeptidyl tRNA from acceptor to donor site

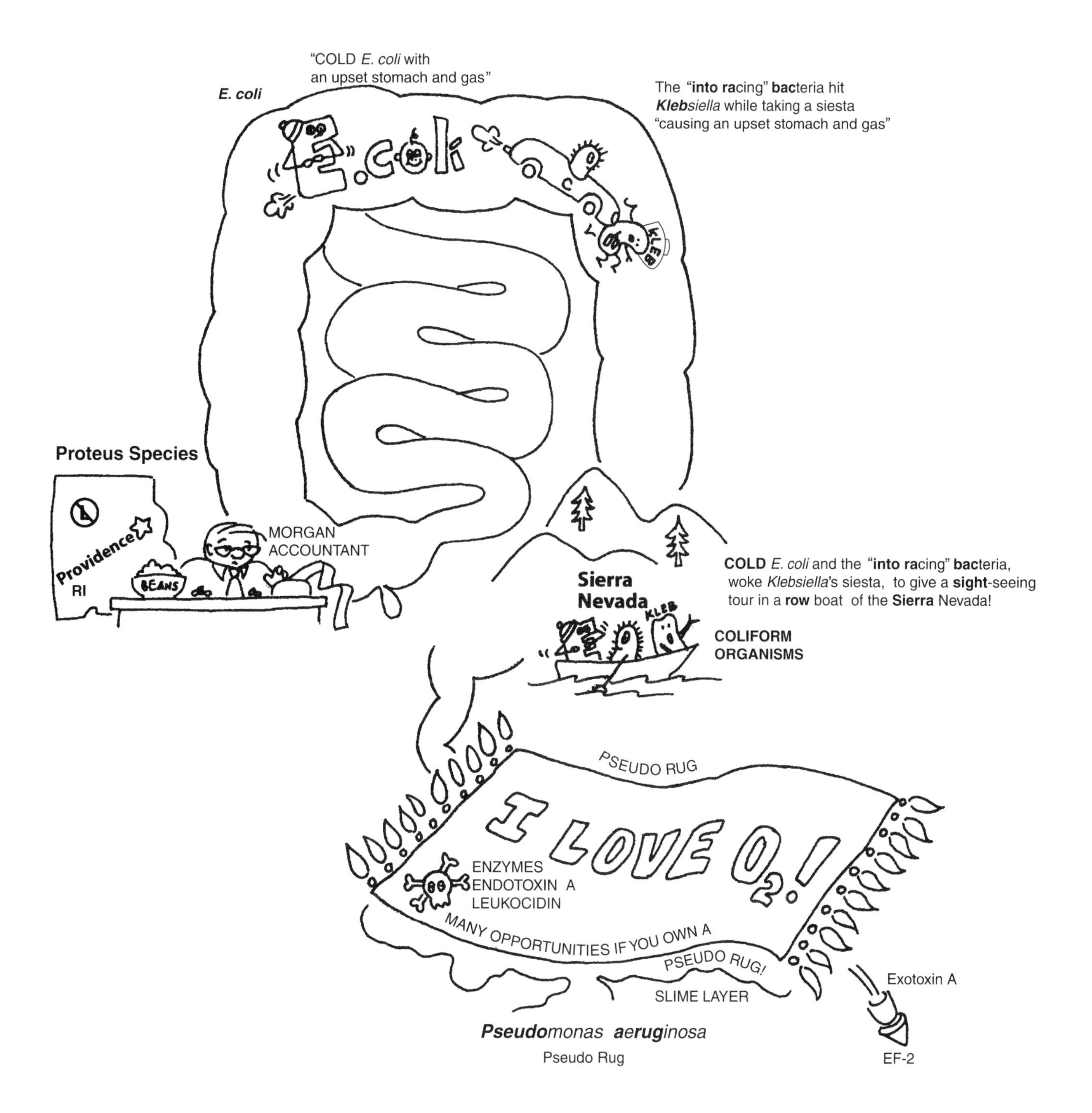
"COLD *E. coli* with
an upset stomach and gas"
E. coli
The "**into ra**cing" **bac**teria hit
Kleb*siella* while taking a siesta
"causing an upset stomach and gas"
E.coli
KLEB
Proteus Species
Providence
RI
BEANS
MORGAN
ACCOUNTANT
Sierra
Nevada
KLEB
COLD *E. coli* and the "**into ra**cing" **bac**teria,
woke *Klebsiella*'s siesta, to give a **sight**-seeing
tour in a **row** boat of the **Sierra** Nevada!
COLIFORM
ORGANISMS
PSEUDO RUG
I LOVE O_2!
ENZYMES
ENDOTOXIN A
LEUKOCIDIN
MANY OPPORTUNITIES IF YOU OWN A
PSEUDO RUG!
SLIME LAYER
Exotoxin A
EF-2
Pseudo*monas* ***aerug****inosa*
Pseudo Rug

NOTES

PRINCIPAL INVASIVE INTESTINAL PATHOGENS THAT PRODUCE DISEASES CONFINED TO INTESTINAL TISSUE

⇒ contained in container

"On a trip to the farm, on Jan. 1957 (it was a hot Sunday), *E. coli* hemorrhaged, after naming a cow Emily."

Enterohemorrhagic *E. coli*

- predominate organism *E. coli* D157:H7
  0157⇒Jan 1957
  H7⇒hot Sunday
- **y**ou **ar**e **Em**ily
  ⇒ hemolytic **urem**ic syndrome
- cow→cattle most common reservoir
- *Shiga*-like cytotoxins or verotoxins
- diagnose by serotyping
- *E. coli* 0157: H7 fails to ferment sorbitol
  ⇒ "cow's **sore butt**"
- causes hemolytic anemia and renal failure
- can get food poisoning from meat that is undercooked

Vibrio parahaemolyticus

⇒ vibrating comma-shaped fish

- halophilic (salt-loving) marine organism inhabiting estuaries
- gastroenteritis→uncooked sea food
- watery diarrhea

Enteroinvasive *E. coli*

⇒ invades

- *Shigella*-like symptoms

***Shigella* Species**

⇒ seagull

"Because of an upset stomach the **disen**chanted **seagull flex**ed for her **son**ny **boy**!"

disenchanted—*S. dysenteriae*
flexed—*S. flexneri*
sonny—*S. sonnei*
boy—*S. boydii*

- upset stomach—acid producing
- no gas
- ferment glucose but not lactose
- do not produce H_2S
- somatic O-antigen
- bacillary dysentery
  ⇒ (bloody) diarrhea
  ⇒ transmissible by food and **water** (*S. **son**nei* type)
  ⇒ "Don't let your **son**s **eat** or **drink** by the **seashore**!"
- organisms reach small intestine to cause diarrhea 48 hrs after ingestion→alarm clock
- to penetrate large intestine required 140 megadalton plasmid
- organism enclosed in vacuole derived from epithelial cell plasma membrane
- cell invasion causes PMN inflammatory response
- produce exotoxin (*Shiga* toxin)→ inactivates 60S→cell death (mostly produced by *S. dysenteriae*)
- bleeding from ulcers
- doesn't enter bloodstream→except in debilitated individuals
- treat with ampicillin

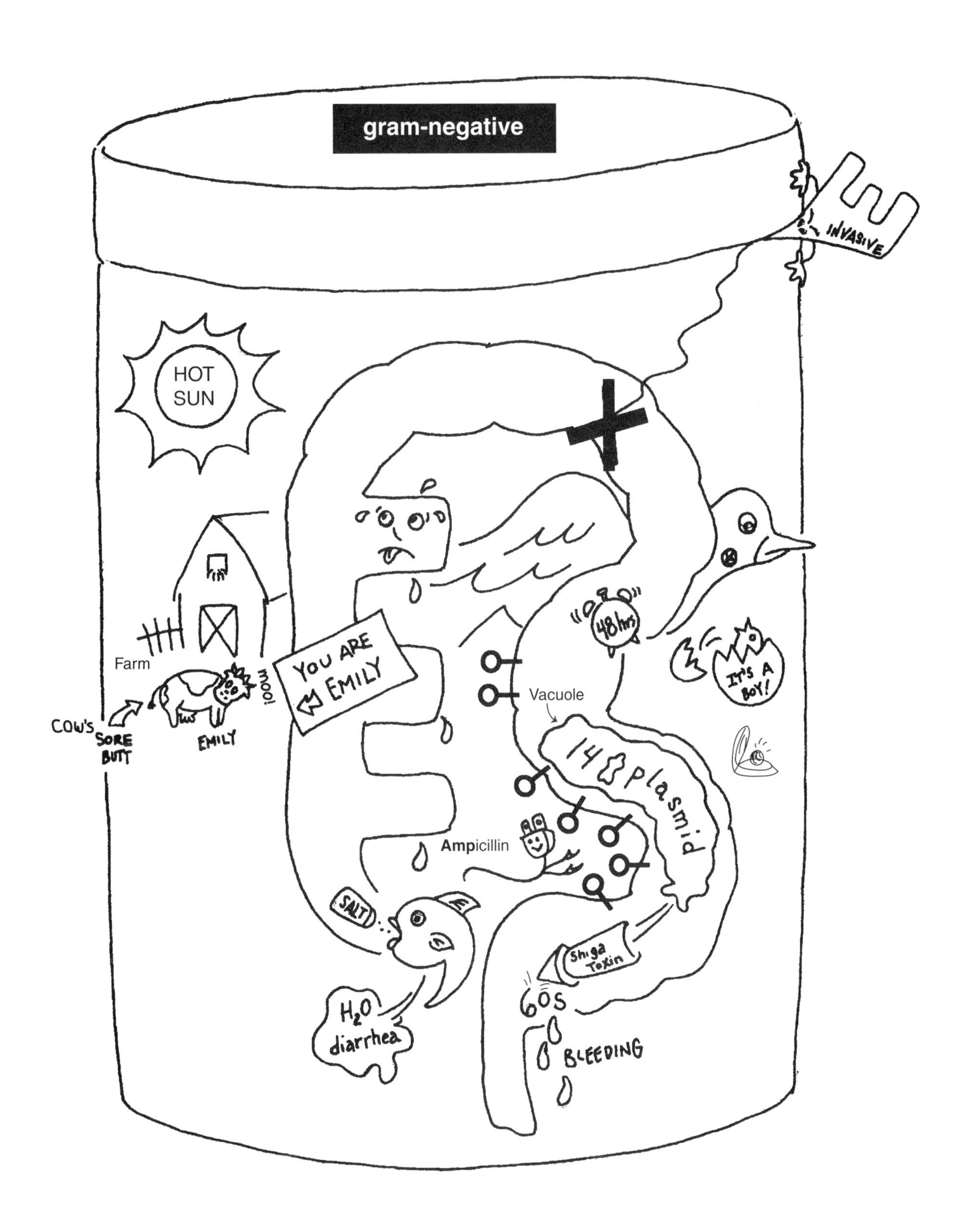
gram-negative
INVASIVE
HOT
SUN
48hrs
YOU ARE
EMILY
Farm
moo!
COW'S
SORE
BUTT
EMILY
IT'S A
BOY!
Vacuole
14 plasmid
Ampicillin
SALT
Shiga
Toxin
60S
H_2O
diarrhea
BLEEDING

NOTES

SALMONELLA

Produce

gas, acid, H_2S

Ferment

glucose but not lactose

Antigens

O, H, Vi, or K for *S. typhi*

Cause

gastroenteritis
enteric fever
septicemia

Exceptions to Drawing

S. typhi
- ⇒ produce acid but no gas
- ⇒ type K—capsular antigen

Species

S. typhi (tie)
S. choleraesuis (call Laura Sue)
S. enteritidis (intestines)

Transmission

- food and water contaminated by infected animals or humans (typhoid/paratyphoid)

Gastroenteritis (Food Poisoning)

- ingesting contaminated food/water
- incubation period 8–24 hrs
- organisms adhere to brush border of epithelial cells of distal ileum and colon and disrupt microvilli
- after penetration into epithelial cells, organisms are enclosed in vacuoles that may coalesce
- organisms migrate through epithelium→ induced PMN leukocyte response→ inflammation
- disease causes fever, abdomen pain, and diarrhea (from mucosal cell invasion and enterotoxin production)
- no antibiotic therapy recommended

Enteric Fever

- contaminated food/H_2O transmission
- *S. typhi* (typhoid fever)
- 1–2 weeks incubation
- initiate macrophage response in lamina propria
- survive in macrophage→travel to mesenteric lymph nodes→enter bloodstream→removed by fixed macrophage
- multiply and re-enter blood
- can produce infection in bone, mesenteric lymph nodes, liver, biliary tract, and spleen
- receding of the intestine with *S. typhi* via bile (causes diarrhea)
- causes: ulceration of Peyer's patches and hemorrhaging, spiking fever and chills
- spleen and liver increase in size

Septicemia

- ⇒ September
- most often caused by *S. choleraesuis*
- similar to enteric fever but no localized intestinal infection

Prevention Important

1) • sanitation
   • pasteurization of milk
   • H_2O treatment
2) immunization with typhoid vaccine

Treatment

- fluid replacement
- treatment of enteric fever and septicemia with antibiotics→chloramphenicol and ampicillin

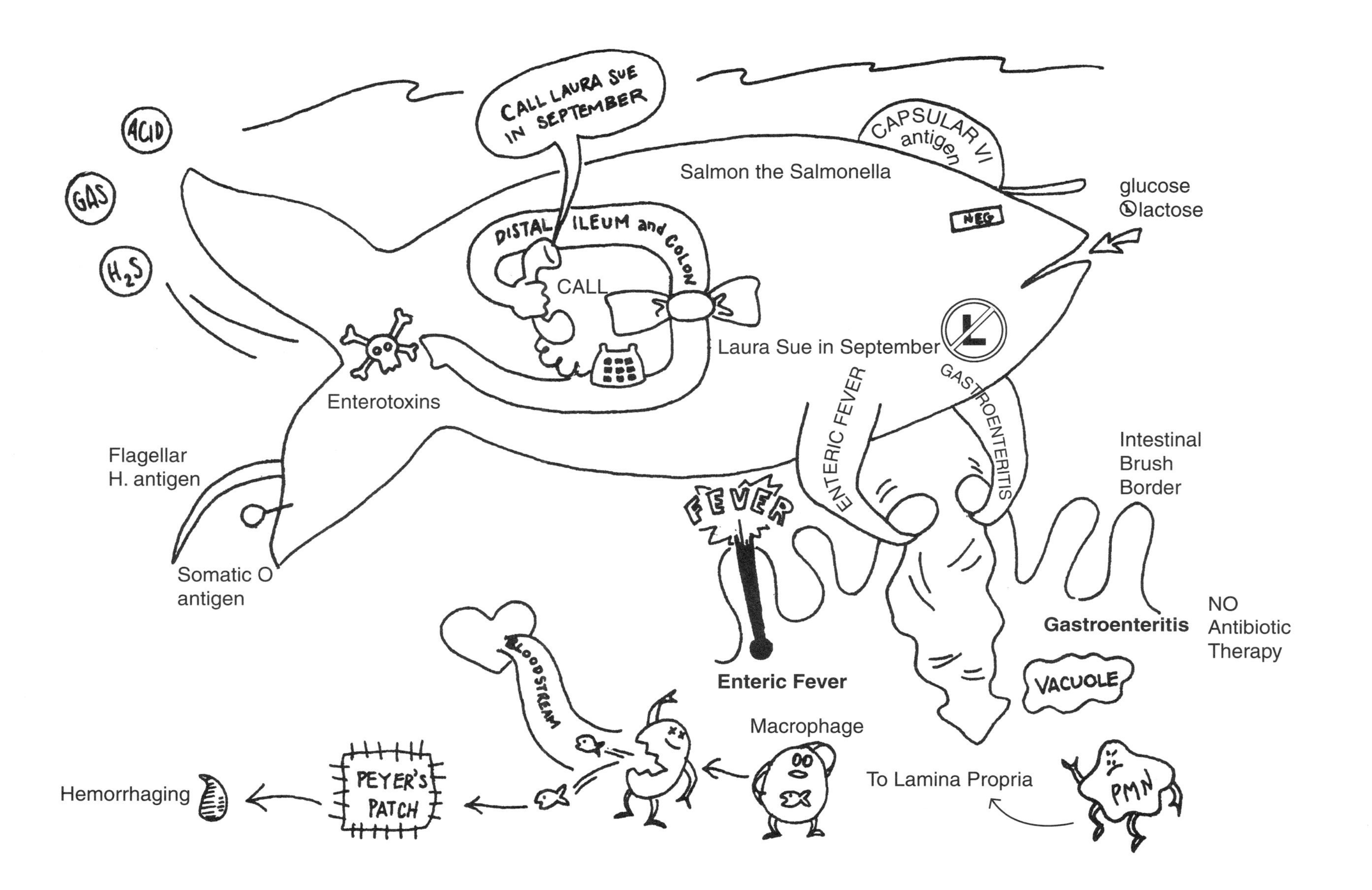
ACID
GAS
H_2S
CALL LAURA SUE IN SEPTEMBER
CAPSULAR VI antigen
Salmon the Salmonella
glucose
lactose
NEG
DISTAL ILEUM and COLON
CALL
Laura Sue in September
Enterotoxins
ENTERIC FEVER
GASTROENTERITIS
Intestinal Brush Border
Flagellar H. antigen
Somatic O antigen
FEVER
NO Antibiotic Therapy
Gastroenteritis
BLOODSTREAM
Enteric Fever
VACUOLE
Macrophage
To Lamina Propria
PMN
Hemorrhaging
PEYER'S PATCH

NOTES

CAMPYLOBACTER JEJUNI, YERSINIA ENTEROCOLITICA, HELICOBACTER PYLORI

Campylobacter jejuni
(Curved Gram-Negative)

⇒ **camp**ing **bac**k pack, **June**

- part of indigenous **flora** (flower) of **mam**mals (mama) and **bird**s
- organisms **invade** small and large intestine
- inflammation, abscess formation and ulceration occur
- some strains produce enterotoxin

Symptoms

- nausea, fever, diarrhea (watery or bloody), severe abdominal pain
- few individuals develop bacteremia
- microaerophilic
  - ⇒ grows best at 5% oxygen (oxygen tank)

Yersinia enterocolitica

⇒ **You're sin**ner
"Tiny sinning bacteria in zoo"

- tiny gram-negative rod which produces enteritis in animals
- acquired from animal carriers⇒(zoo)
- similar disease to *C. jejuni*

Helicobacter pylori

⇒ **Helico**pter **Pie**

- resembles *C. jejuni* morphologically and biochemically
- motile⇒(helicopter form of transportation)
- causes chronic gastritis, gastric and duodenal ulcers⇒(x's on stomach and duodenum)
- selectively adheres to gastric mucosal cells after penetrating mucus
- generates urease→survive acidic stomach
- generates ammonia→cytotoxic to gastric epithelial cells

Treatment

- bismuth (bismuth or bust), metronidazole (metro), amoxicillin (**A mo**m **ox** is **sill**y!), tetracycline (tetracycle)

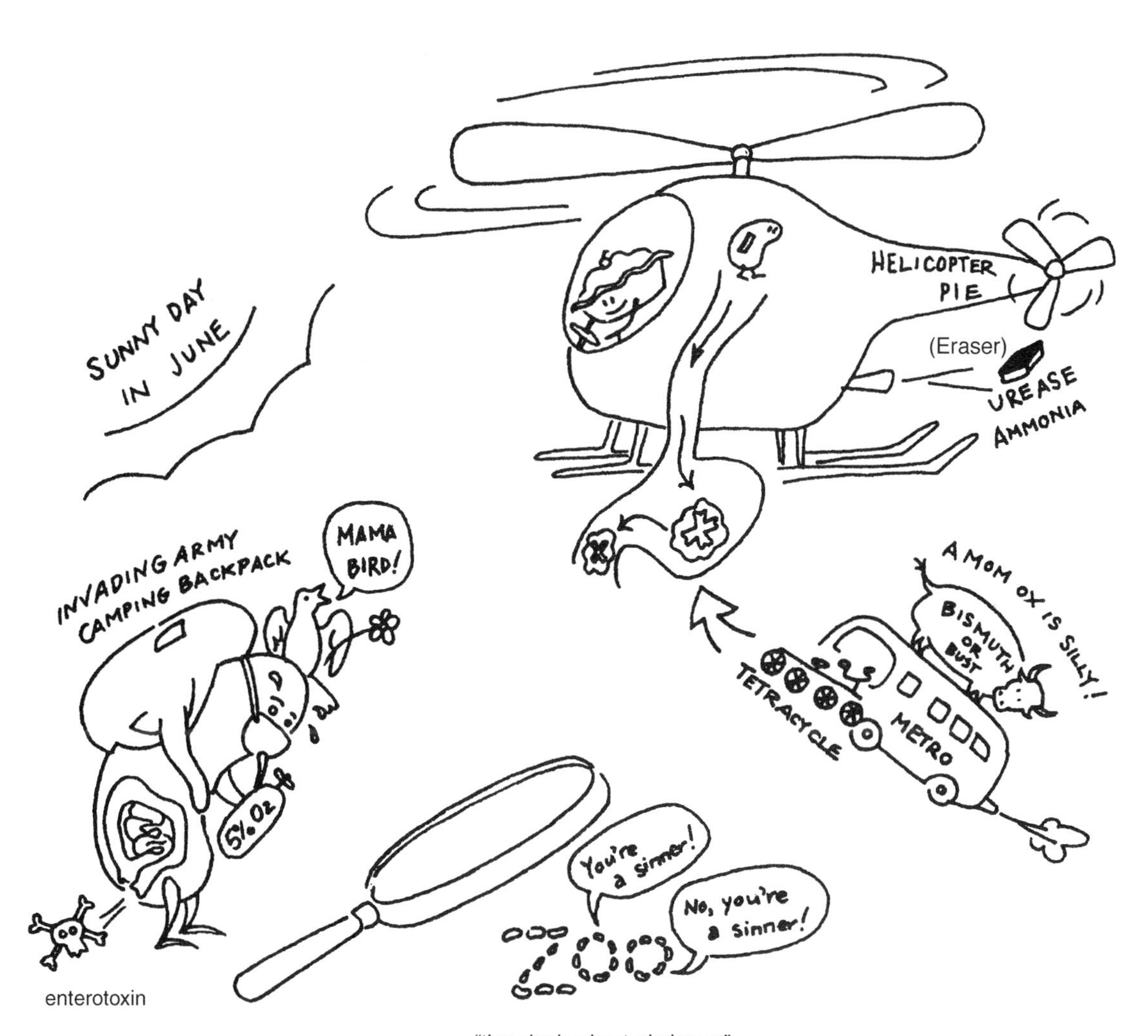

"tiny sinning bacteria in zoo"

NOTES

NEISSERIA

⇒ (Nice Sara from Syria)
- small gram-negative cocci
- non-spore-forming
  ⇒ no s'more
- non-flagellated
- family Veillonellaceae
  ⇒ anaerobic gram-negative cocci ($\not{O}_2$)
- pathogens—*N. gonorrhoeae* and *N. meningitidis*

NEISSERIA GONORRHOEAE

⇒ Gone is Rhea
- human only natural host

Mode of Transmission

- sexual intercourse
- oral-genital contact
- rectal intercourse
- contaminated inanimate objects (uncommon)

Virulence Factors

- endotoxin→lipopolysaccharide (LPS)
- Pili, IgA protease, capsule clinical manifestations

Clinical Manifestations

- inoculation→urethra and/or cervix
- superficial epithelial penetration
- genitourinary tract involvement
  ♂ symptomatic-pus
  ♂ asymptomatic
- disseminated gonococcal infection (DGI)
  ⇒ invade bloodstream
  ⇒ arthritis, dermatitis, endocarditis, pericarditis, perihepatitis (Fitz-Hugh-Curtis syndrome)
- gonococcal ophthalmia neonatorum
  ⇒ Crede's treatment: 1–2% silver nitrate instilled into eyes
- conjunctivitis in adults; vulvovaginitis

Diagnosis

- Gram stain, culture (chocolate agar, Thayer Martin medium)

Treatment

- ciprofloxacin, ofloxacin, cefixime, ceftriaxone
- no vaccine

KINGELLA

⇒ King
⇒ normal flora of upper respiratory tract (nose)
⇒ endocarditis (♡)

MORAXELLA

⇒ (no more wax)
⇒ normal flora of nasopharynx (nose)
⇒ infection in compromised hosts→ *Moraxella catarrhalis*
⇒ cause otitis media (ear) and pneumonia (lung)

ACINTOBACTER CALCO-ACETICUS

⇒ (a sign on back)
⇒ normal flora of upper respiratory
⇒ cause hospital-acquired pneumonia
⇒ (man pointing to lungs)

NEISSERIA MENINGITIDIS

⇒ Many giants
- primary cause of cerebrospinal meningitis
- transmission→nasopharyngeal secretions

Virulence Factors

- LPS, capsule, IgA protease (claw on skull)
- serogroups—based on polysaccharide capsule
- serotypes—outer membrane proteins
- immunotype—LPS

Treatment

- penicillin ⇒ penny
- chemoprophylaxis: vaccine ( ) or rifamycin ( )

King
"NO MORE WAX!"
A sign on back
HOSPITAL
NICE
SARA
from SYRIA
gram-negative
"Gone is Rhea, she needs some CO_2 and glucose."
CAPSULE
RHEA PERLMAN
LPS
PILI
IgA Protease
=
SKIP
-ciprofloxacin
IgA
IgA
IgA
Many Giants
N. meningitidis
cerebral meningitis
Treatment
ONE CENT
Penny Chemo-prophylaxis
IgA
LPS
RIF
rifamycin or vaccine
NOSE

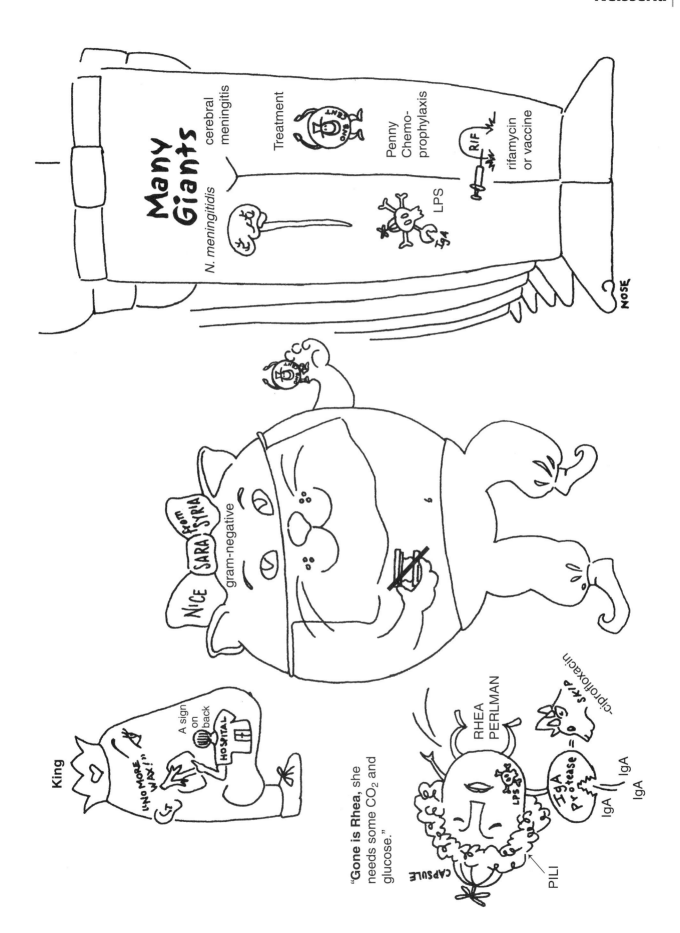

NOTES

HAEMOPHILUS

⇒ means "blood loving," hence RBC

***Haemophilus*⇒RBC in Drawing**

- part of normal flora of upper respiratory (nose) tract & oral cavity
- small gram-negative bacilli
- non-motile; non-spore-forming (⊄)
- fastidious growth requirements
- hemophilic nature→biosynthesis of one or two substances present in RBCs
  X-factor: heat-stable; hemin
  V-factor: heat-labile; NAD
  ⇒ V, X factor factory
- satellite phenomenon
- staphylcocci excrete V-factor into medium and will support the growth of *Haemophilus* species requiring this factor on media deficient in the V-factor

H. influenzae
Subtype *Aegyptius*

⇒ camel
- transmission via contaminated objects that contact face and eyes
  ⇒ hand towel

Pathogenesis

- conjunctivitis (eye) or Brazilian purpuric fever

Laboratory Diagnosis

⇒ laboratory microscope
- chocolate agar
- immunofluorescence
- Quellung reaction

Immunity

⇒ I am a moon!
- anticapsular antibodies
- somatic antigens induce complement
  ⇒ some ADDICT!

Treatment

- chloramphenicol + ampicillin; rifampin for chemoprophylaxis

H. parainfluenzae* and *H. influenzae

⇒ In Flew Enza
- mostly found in children
- transmission: person to person by respiratory tract
- virulence factors
  ⇒ polysaccharide capsule→protects against phagocytosis→most strains causing meningitis are serotype b (Bon witch's hat)
  ⇒ IgA protease

Pathogenesis

- nasopharyngeal colonization
  ⇒ nasopharyngitis major symptom
- direct extension of organism from site of colonization
  ⇒ sinusitis, otitis media
  bronchitis, pneumonia
- local tissue invasion
  ⇒ epiglotitis→potentially lethal when obstruction occurs
  ⇒ pericarditis
  ⇒ facial cellulitis
- bacteremia
  ⇒ meningitis→children
  ⇒ endocarditis
  ⇒ brain abscess
  ⇒ arthritis
  ⇒ osteomyelitis

H. ducreyi

- transmission
  ⇒ sexual contact
- causes ulcerative disease→chancroid
- chancroid formation (soft chance) at the site of inoculation
- treatment with erythromycin (this is eery!) or ceftriaxone

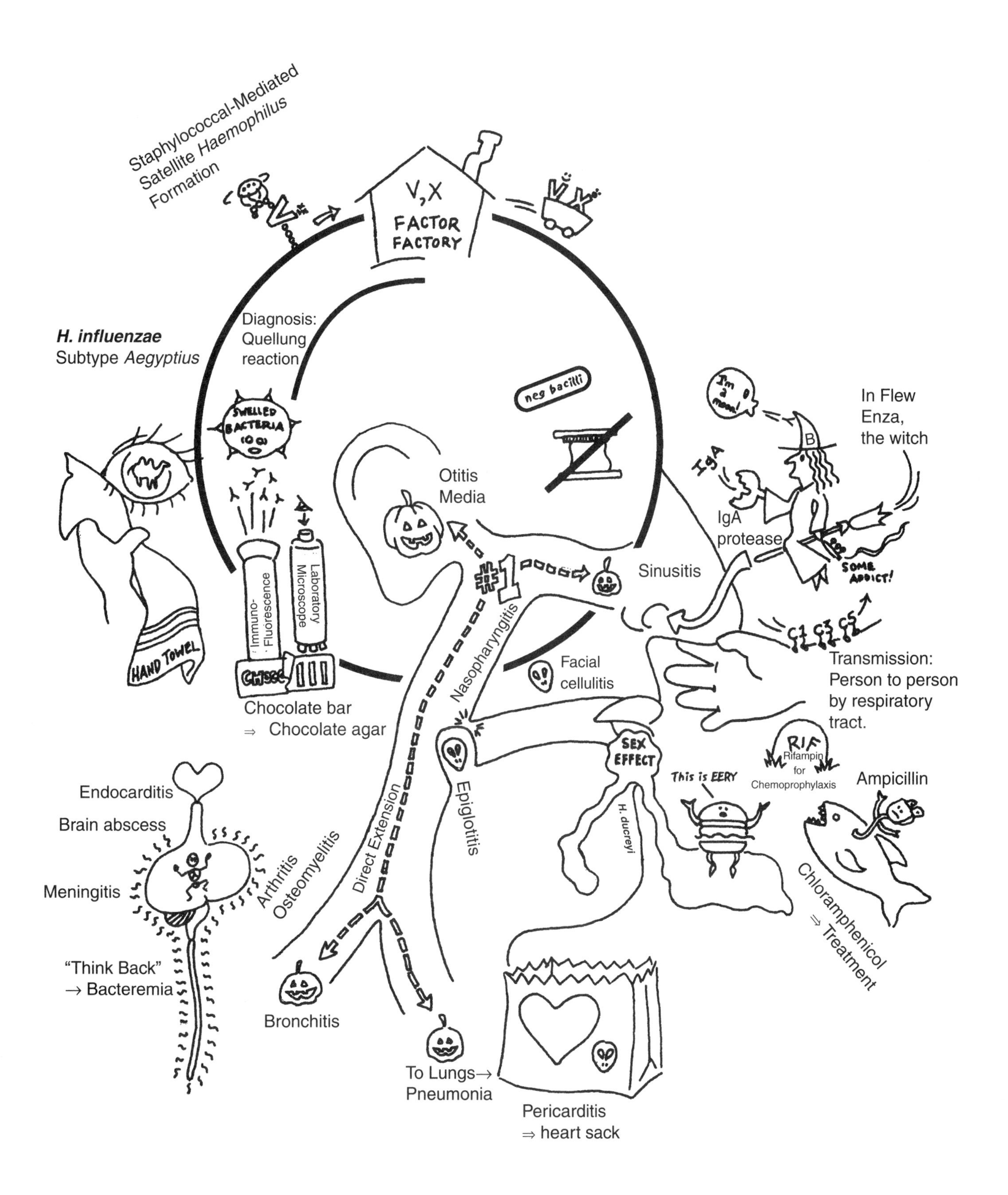
Staphylococcal-Mediated Satellite Haemophilus Formation
V,X
FACTOR FACTORY
Diagnosis: Quellung reaction
H. influenzae
Subtype Aegyptius
SWELLED BACTERIA
neg bacilli
Otitis Media
Immuno-Fluorescence
Laboratory Microscope
HAND TOWEL
Chocolate bar ⇒ Chocolate agar
#1
Sinusitis
Nasopharyngitis
Facial cellulitis
I'm a moon!
In Flew Enza, the witch
IgA
IgA protease
SOME ADDICT!
C1 C3 C5
Transmission: Person to person by respiratory tract.
SEX EFFECT
H. ducreyi
This is EERY
RIF
Rifampin for Chemoprophylaxis
Ampicillin
Epiglottitis
Direct Extension
Endocarditis
Brain abscess
Meningitis
Arthritis
Osteomyelitis
"Think Back" → Bacteremia
Bronchitis
To Lungs→ Pneumonia
Pericarditis ⇒ heart sack
Chloramphenicol ⇒ Treatment

OTHER *HAEMOPHILUS* SPECIES

H. paraphrophilus

- ⇒ pair of afros
- causes endocarditis
  - ⇒ ♡

H. haemolyticus

- ⇒ hem lysing
- respiratory tract infections
  - ⇒ Lung

H. aphrophilus

- ⇒ afro on filing cabinet
- causes meningitis (brain) septicemia (SEPT)

Gardnerella vaginalis

- ⇒ (Garden)
- female genital tract infections
- neonatal sepsis (👶)
- clue cells(?)→epithelial cells to which many gram-negative (⊖) coccobacilli (O) are attached

Treatment

- Aminoglycosides
  - ⇒ a mean Geico insurance agent
- tetracycline
  - ⇒ tetracycle
- chloramphenicol
  - ⇒ colorful fin

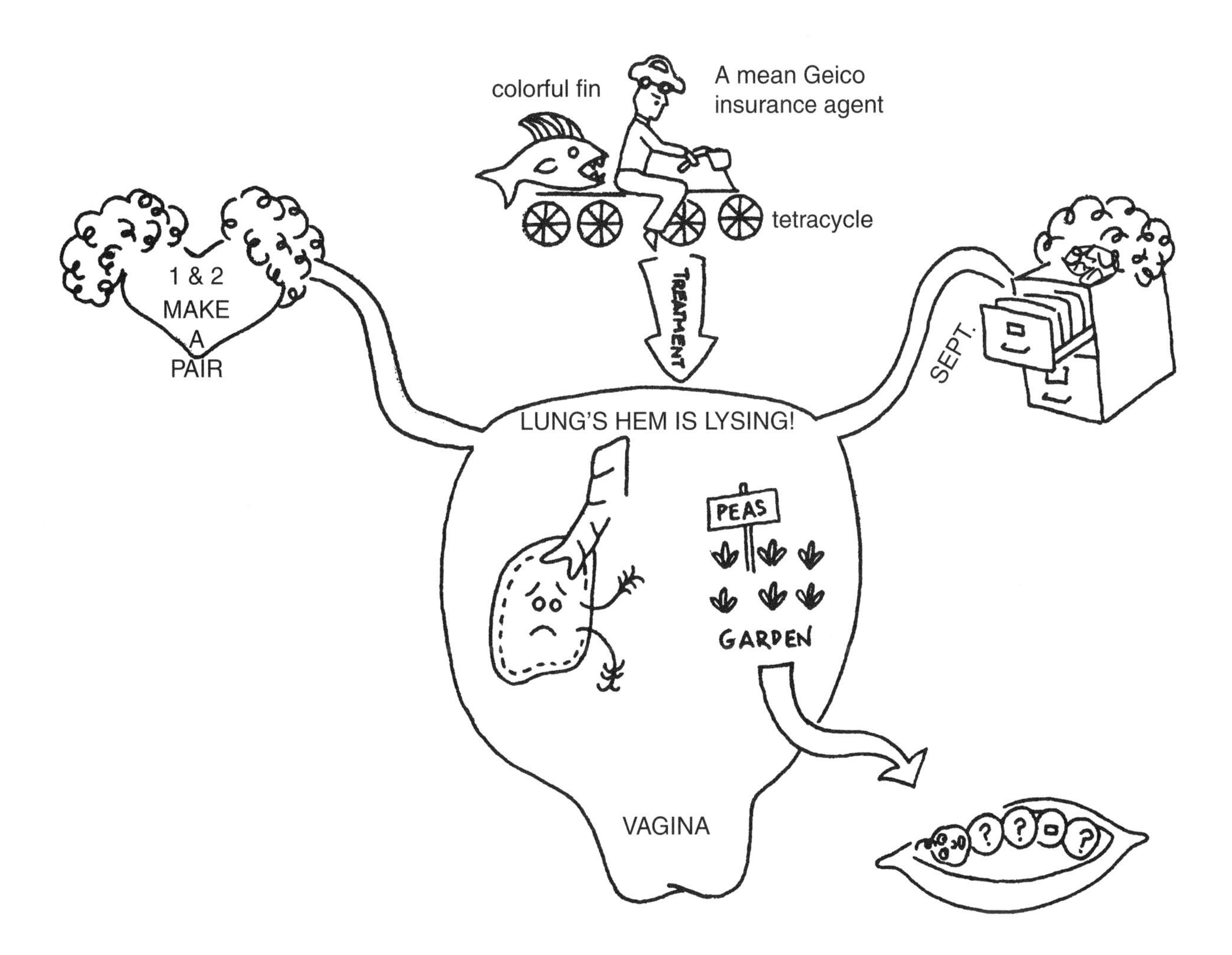
colorful fin
A mean Geico insurance agent
tetracycle
TREATMENT
1 & 2 MAKE A PAIR
SEPT.
LUNG'S HEM IS LYSING!
PEAS
GARDEN
VAGINA

TREPONEMA PALLIDUM (SYPHILIS)

⇒ Trippin' Ema on a palindrome and silly Phyllis (syphilis)

Modes of Infection

- sexual contact (condoms), congenitally acquired (baby), blood transfusion (IV bag), direct inoculation ("wants to touch you")

Pathogenesis

⇒ picture contains explanation

Congenital Syphilis (Baby)

- pregnant women with 1°, 2°, 3° syphilis
  - ⇒ 15th to 18th weeks of gestation
  - ⇒ treponemes infect placenta and pass into fetal circulation
- several clinical manifestations are possible
  a. free from disease
  b. late abortion
  c. stillborn: pneumonia alba→lungs are grayish white, incompletely developed and fill entire thoracic cavity
  d. death shortly after birth
  e. neonatal disease after birth
     - lesions primarily on mucocutaneous membranes and bones—any organ can be involved
     - neurosyphilis

Neurosyphilis

- asymptomatic
- symptomatic (3 clinical manifestations)
  1) **meningovascular:** inflammation of meninges and blood vessels
  2) parenchymatous: destruction of nerve cells
     - ⇒ general paresis—brain involvement
     - ⇒ tabes dorsalis—spinal cord involvement

Late Benign Syphilis ⇒ (Blind ⚕)

- formation of non-specific granulomatous (granule mat) lesions (gumma) which can involve any organ

Laboratory Diagnosis

- not diagnosed by isolation and identification of organism
- three means of diagnosing syphilis
  1) clinical manifestations
  2) direct demonstration of organism
  3) serological tests
     - nonspecific nontreponemal reaginic Ab
       - ⇒ reagin (Wassermann)
       - ⇒ cardiolipin

Treatment

- penicillin is antimicrobial of choice (penny)
- treat if exposed in last 3 months
- Jarisch-Herxheimer reaction (Jar)
  - ⇒ systemic reaction occurring 1 to 2 hrs after initial treatment with antibiotics due to endotoxin release by lysed spirochetes

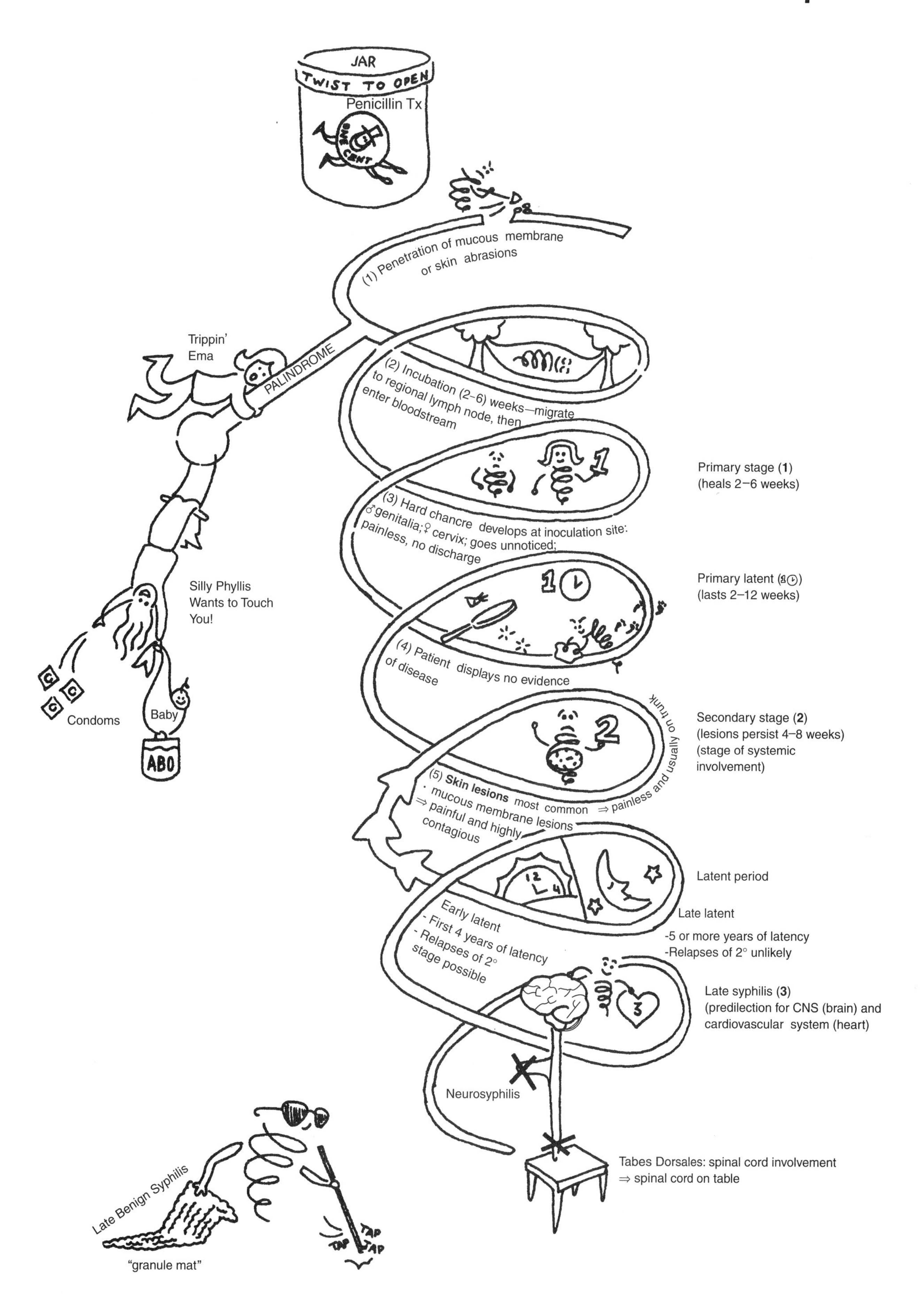
JAR
TWIST TO OPEN
Penicillin Tx
ONE CENT
(1) Penetration of mucous membrane or skin abrasions
Trippin' Ema
PALINDROME
(2) Incubation (2–6) weeks—migrate to regional lymph node, then enter bloodstream
Primary stage (1)
(heals 2–6 weeks)
(3) Hard chancre develops at inoculation site: ♂ genitalia; ♀ cervix; goes unnoticed; painless, no discharge
Silly Phyllis Wants to Touch You!
Primary latent
(lasts 2–12 weeks)
(4) Patient displays no evidence of disease
Condoms
Baby
ABO
Secondary stage (2)
(lesions persist 4–8 weeks)
(stage of systemic involvement)
(5) **Skin lesions** most common ⇒ painless and usually on trunk
· mucous membrane lesions ⇒ painful and highly contagious
Latent period
Late latent
-5 or more years of latency
-Relapses of 2° unlikely
Early latent
- First 4 years of latency
- Relapses of 2° stage possible
Late syphilis (3)
(predilection for CNS (brain) and cardiovascular system (heart)
Neurosyphilis
Tabes Dorsales: spinal cord involvement
⇒ spinal cord on table
Late Benign Syphilis
"granule mat"
TAP
TAP
TAP

NOTES

NONVENEREAL TREPONEMATOSES

- group of 3 contagious diseases endemic among rural populations of tropical and subtropical populations
- classification of organisms primarily based on disease manifestations

Diagnosis

- demonstration of organism in early lesions

Treatment

- penicillin (penny)

Treponema carateum (Pinto)

⇒ karate team ⇒ "pinto"

Transmission

- direct contact with open skin lesions
- common in children before puberty

Pathogenesis: Skin Lesions

- skin lesions initially appear around site of initial inoculation
- later skin lesions occur over entire body→ frequently involve wrists, elbows, ankles
- does not impair general health but is disfiguring
- "Sippin' high Listerine"

Treponema syphilis

- var. endemic syphilis (bejel)→"bee with gel in hair"

Transmission

- mucosal inoculation
- direct contact: biting, kissing, breastfeeding
- indirect contact: sharing drinking and eating utensils, tooth picks, tobacco pipes

Pathogenesis

- mucous membrane, cutaneous, and bone involvement
- primary lesion at site of inoculation
- secondary cutaneous lesions over entire body
- late granulomatous lesions of skin, nasopharynx, and bones

Treponema pertenue (yaws)

Transmission

- direct contact with open skin lesions
- common in children before puberty

Pathogenesis

- skin lesions appear around initial site of invasion
- bone lesions occur later involving skull, sternum, tibia, and other bones

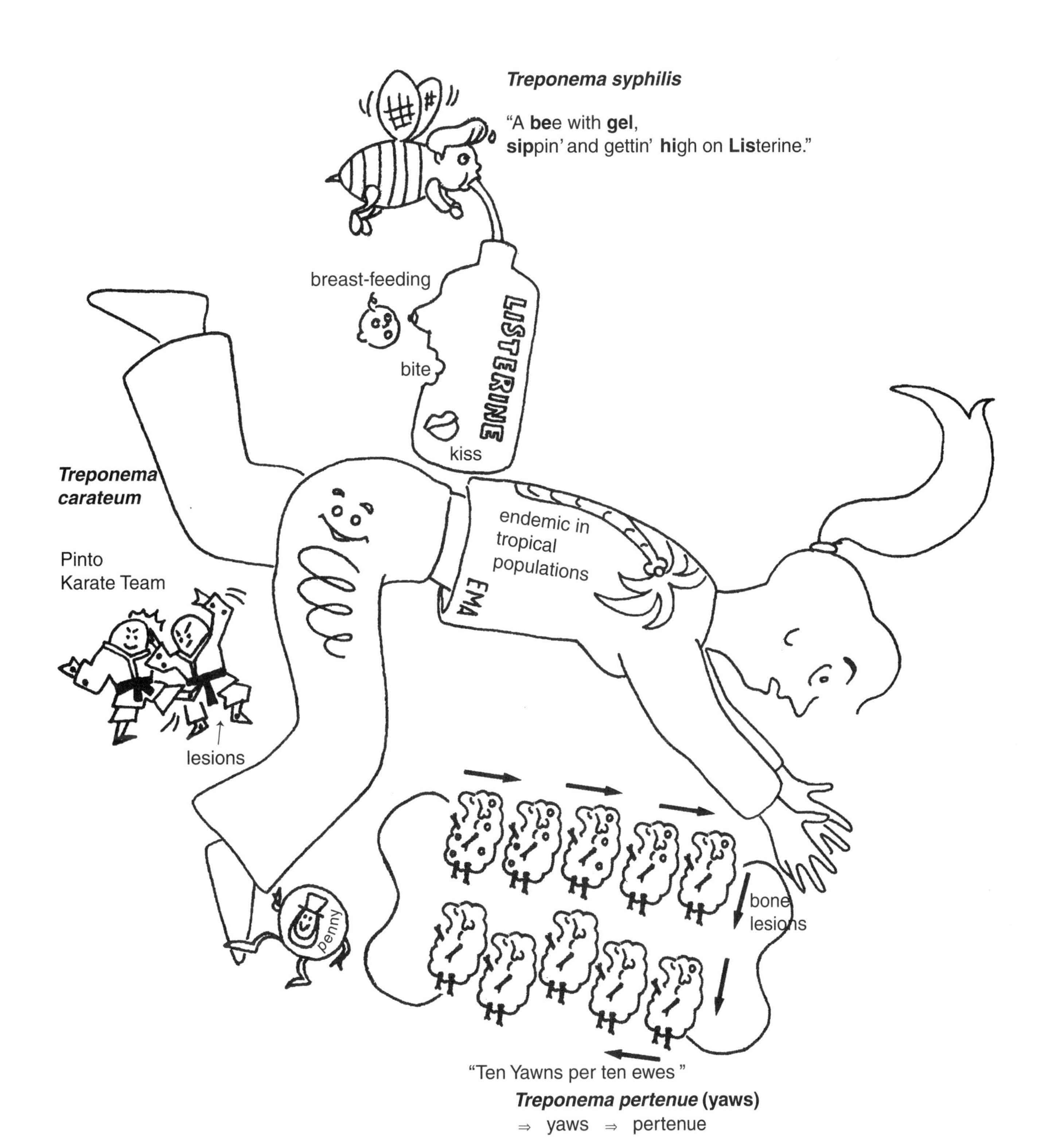

***Treponema pertenue* (yaws)**

⇒ yaws ⇒ pertenue

NOTES

BORRELIA

⇒ barrel

BORRELIA

Pathogenesis

- inoculation followed by incubation period of 4 to 18 days
- febrile illness: sudden onset of fever→ *Borrelia* can be recovered from blood
- afebrile period: no symptom→no *Borrelia* in blood
- usually 3–10 relapses
- mechanism of relapse *Borrelia*→bactericidal antibodies→ recovery→*Borrelia* sequestered into internal organs→next febrile episode due to invasion of bloodstream of spirochetes antigenically different from preceding febrile period→ultimate recovery due to antibody formation against several antigenic types

Diagnosis

- *Borrelia* in blood of febrile patients

Treatment

- tetracycline (tetracycle)

RELAPSING FEVER

⇒ caused by several species of spirochetes (⸘) of the genus *Borrelia* (barrel) and characterized clinically by alternating periods of febrile illness with apparent recovery

Transmission (louse and tick)

- louse-borne relapsing fever (*Borrelia recurrentis*)
  - ⇒ "current"
  - ⇒ also called endemic relapsing fever
  - ⇒ human body louse ingests blood of infected individual
  - ⇒ *B. recurrentis* multiplies in hemolymph of louse
  - ⇒ louse crushed on susceptible individual resulting in organism release
- tick-borne relapsing fever
  (*Borrelia hermsii*)⇒("Her MS II)
  (*Borrelia turicatae*)⇒("tumicate on tick")
  - ⇒ also called endemic relapsing fever
  - ⇒ tick ingests blood of infected rodent (primarily ground squirrels and prairie dogs)
  - ⇒ *Borrelia* multiplies in all tissues of tick
  - ⇒ during subsequent feeding on susceptible human, tick salivates and defecates, resulting in release of *Borrelia*

FUSOSPIROCHETOSIS—"FUSE ON SPIRAL"

- symbiotic disease involving two microorganisms which are normal flora of oral cavity:
  1) *Borrelia vincentii*⇒(**Vincent** Van Gogh)
  2) fusobacterium⇒(Fuse)
- initiating event: poor oral hygiene or oral injury
- no person-to-person transmission

Pathogenesis

- ulceromembranous stomatitis (John Stomatis)—grayish white pseudomembrane forms in throat
  - ⇒ Vincent's angina—throat and tonsils become ulcerated with extensive tissue damage
- ulcerative gingivostomatitis (gingivitis)—gums/mouth; "trench mouth"→foul odor→ also ANUG (Acute Necrotizing Ulcerative Gingivostomatitis)

Diagnosis

- stained smear of lesion

Treatment

1) tetracycline—Penicillin
2) correct underlying condition

LYME DISEASE

⇒ Lyme
(B. burgdorferi)

⇒ picking his nose

Clinical Manifestations

- 1st stage of disease
  - ⇒ skin lesions—erythema chronicum migrans (ECM) (◎)
  - ⇒ joint stiffness, headache, stiff neck, fever
- 2nd stage
  - ⇒ multiple skin patches, arthritis, neurologic and cardiac manifestations
- 3rd stage of disease
  - ⇒ arthritis, neurologic symptoms

Treatment

- early: doxycycline or amoxicillin; late: ceftriaxone

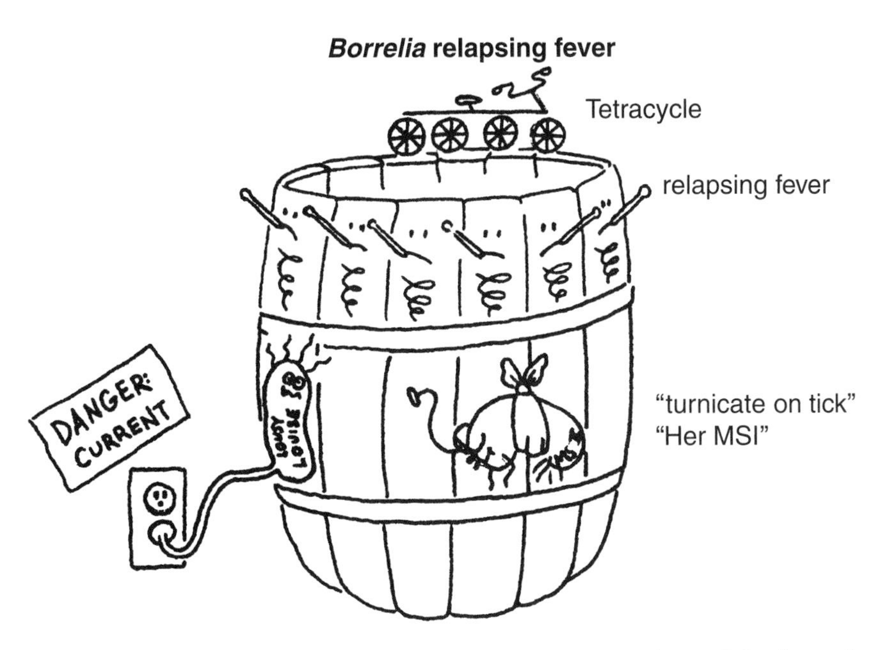
Borrelia relapsing fever
Tetracycle
relapsing fever
"turnicate on tick"
"Her MSI"
DANGER:
CURRENT

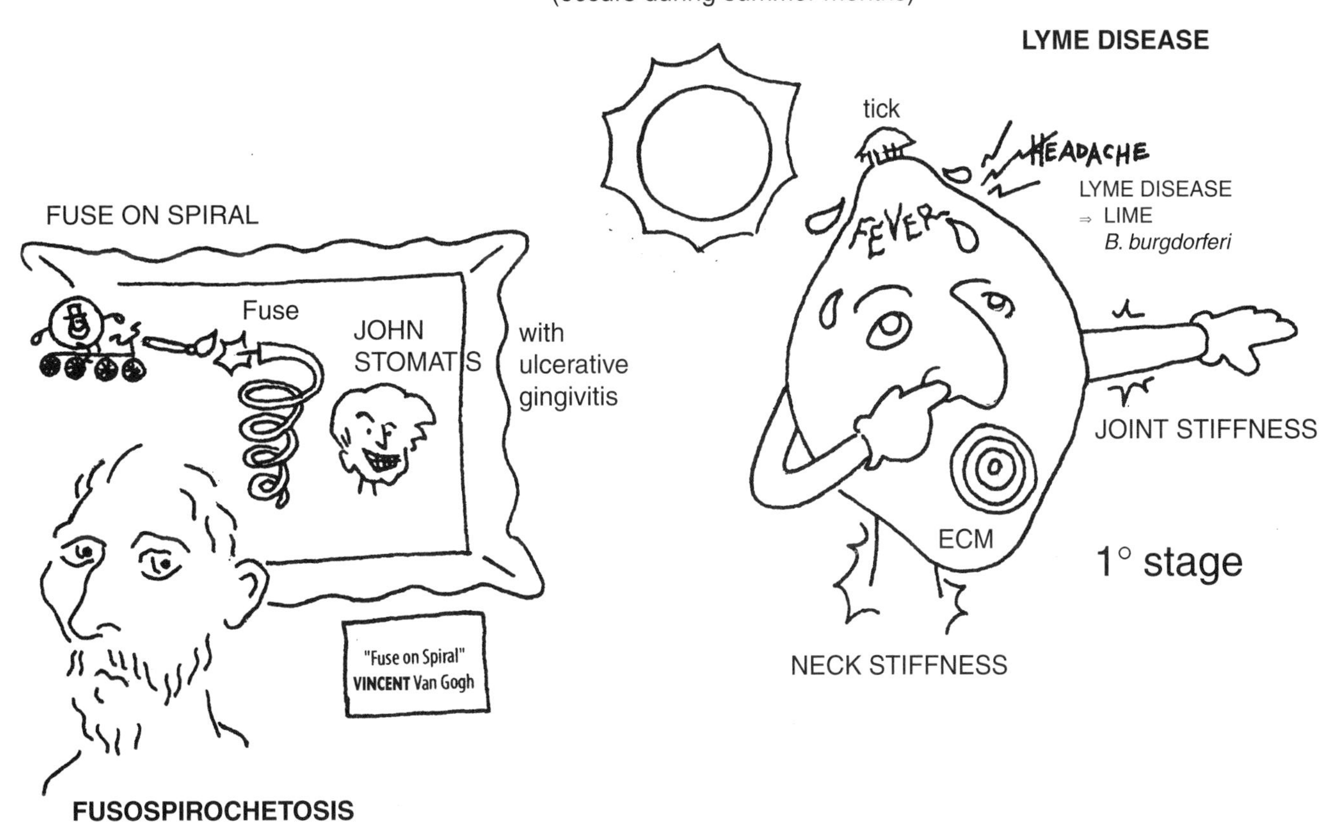
June, July, August
(occurs during summer months)
LYME DISEASE
tick
HEADACHE
LYME DISEASE
⇒ LIME
B. burgdorferi
FEVER
JOINT STIFFNESS
ECM
1° stage
NECK STIFFNESS
FUSE ON SPIRAL
Fuse
JOHN
STOMATIS
with
ulcerative
gingivitis
"Fuse on Spiral"
VINCENT Van Gogh
FUSOSPIROCHETOSIS

LEPTOSPIROSIS

⇒ legs leap

- all leptospira belong to one of two species
  1) *L. interrogans*⇒"being interrogated"
     ⇒ parasitic form
  2) *L. biflexa*—no disease
- found in kidneys and urine of dogs, cats, livestock, and rodents
- excreted profusely in urine

Transmission

- contact with infected or contaminated substance which humans acquire through abraded skin and mucous membranes
- humans dead end host

Pathogenesis

- After penetration of skin and invasion of blood stream
  1) Subclinical Leptospirosis
     ⇒ inapparent infection
  2) Anicteric Leptospirosis
- 1st stage: abrupt onset of fever, muscle pains, and malaise
- afebrile stage
- 2nd stage: many clinical manifestations
  1) Ft. Bragg fever (pre-tibial fever) rash over shins
  2) swineherd's disease—aseptic meningitis
  3) conjunctivitis

3) Icteric Leptospirosis
- 1st stage: same as anicteric
- afebrile
- 2nd stage: impaired renal and hepatic function
- immunity after recovery is lifelong

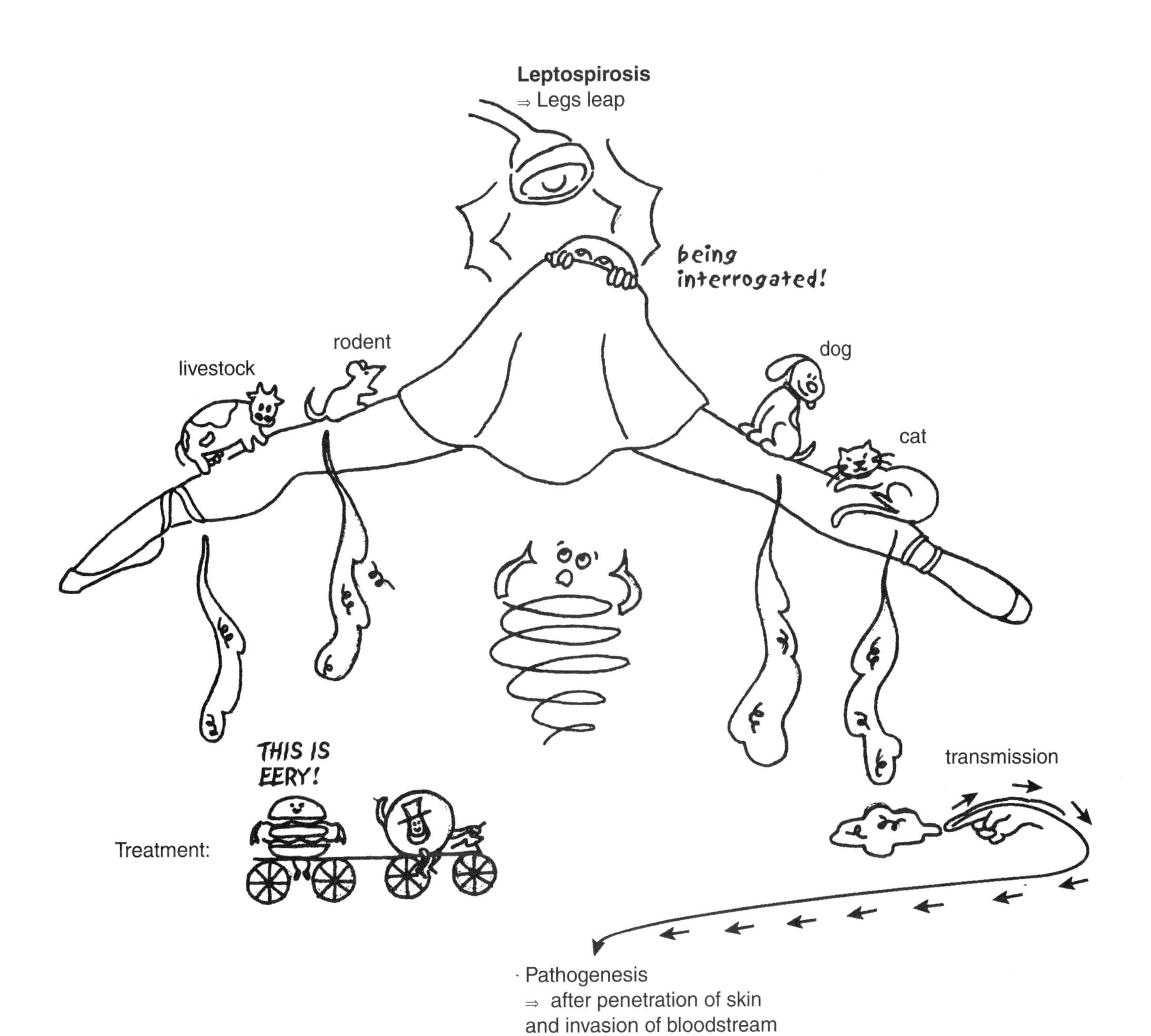

- Pathogenesis
  ⇒ after penetration of skin and invasion of bloodstream

1) Subclinical leptospirosis
   - inapparent infection
2) Anticteric leptospirosis
3) Icteric leptospirosis
   ⇒ severe form of disease

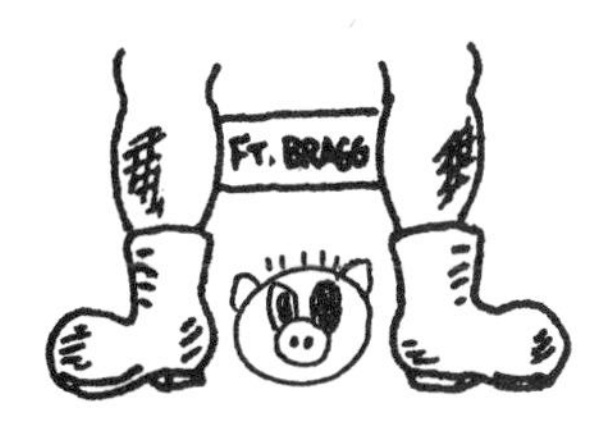

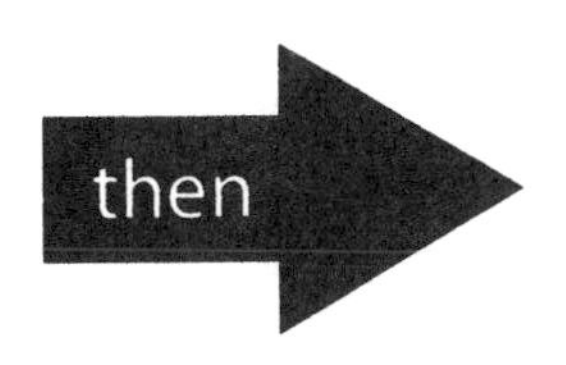

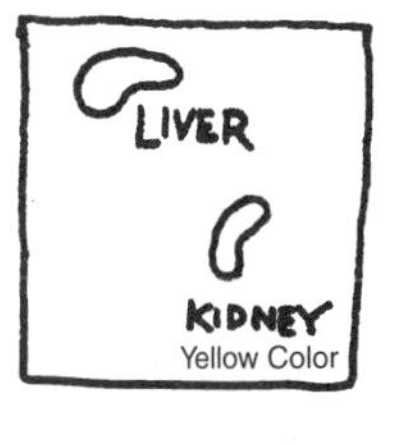

- Weil's syndrome, infectious jaundice

NOTES

YERSINIA

⇒ Your Sin

short, gram-negative bacilli, non-spore-forming

Transmission

1) interruption of rodent-flea-rodent cycle
2) handling of infected animal tissue
3) inhalation of organism—droplets from patient with pneumonia
4) laboratory acquired

Murine Toxin

⇒ (marine fish)

- heat-labile exotoxin primarily responsible for death (fish dressed as death)
- acts on peripheral vascular system

Treatment

- streptomycin, tetracycline, chloramphenicol

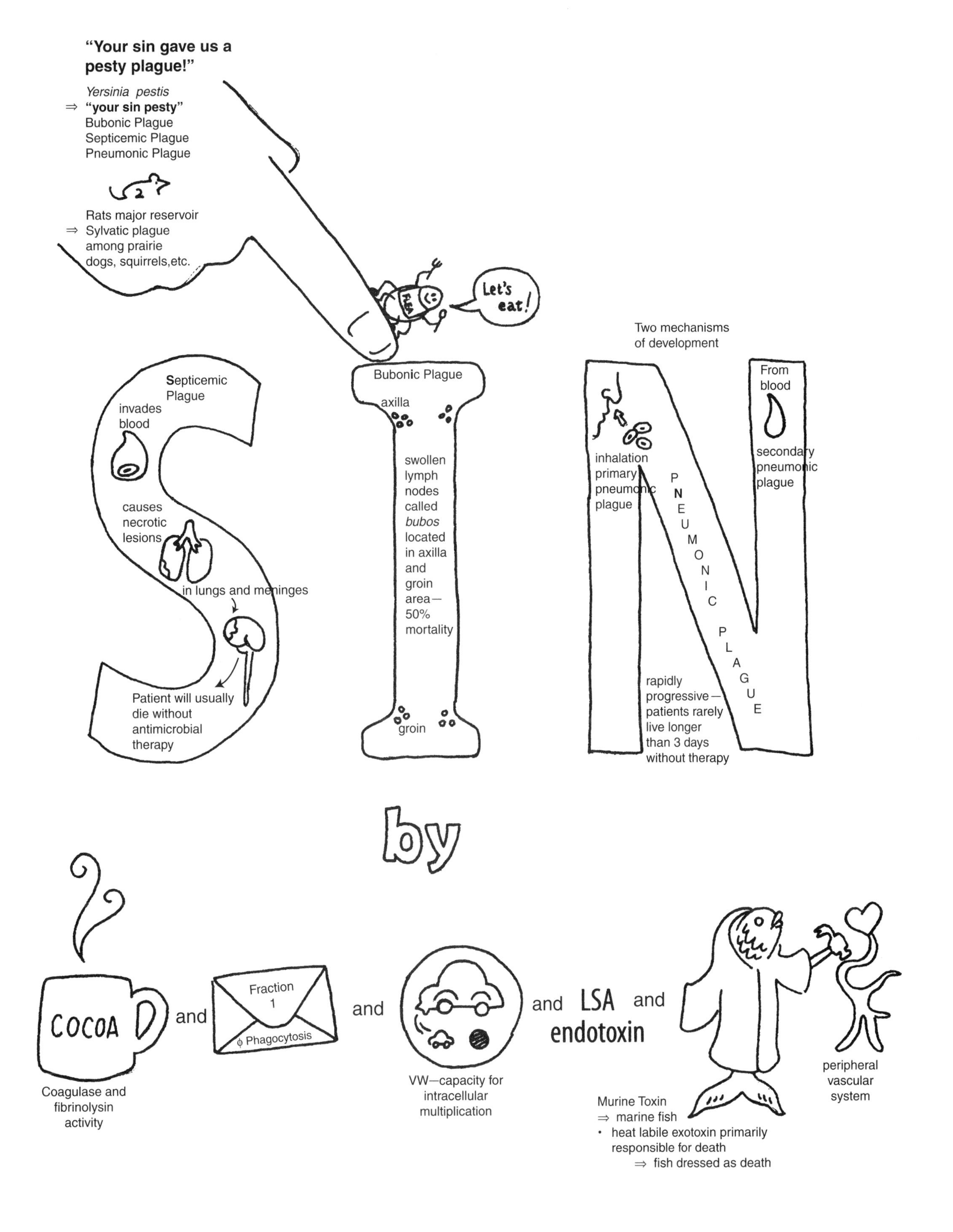
"Your sin gave us a pesty plague!"
Yersinia pestis
⇒ "your sin pesty"
Bubonic Plague
Septicemic Plague
Pneumonic Plague
Rats major reservoir
⇒ Sylvatic plague among prairie dogs, squirrels,etc.
Let's eat!
FLEA
Septicemic Plague
invades blood
causes necrotic lesions
in lungs and meninges
Patient will usually die without antimicrobial therapy
Bubonic Plague
axilla
swollen lymph nodes called bubos located in axilla and groin area—50% mortality
groin
Two mechanisms of development
inhalation primary pneumonic plague
From blood
secondary pneumonic plague
PNEUMONIC PLAGUE
rapidly progressive—patients rarely live longer than 3 days without therapy
by
COCOA
Coagulase and fibrinolysin activity
and
Fraction 1
ϕ Phagocytosis
and
VW—capacity for intracellular multiplication
and LSA and endotoxin
Murine Toxin
⇒ marine fish
• heat labile exotoxin primarily responsible for death
⇒ fish dressed as death
peripheral vascular system

NOTES

⇒ France ⇒ tulip

FRANCISELLA TULARENSIS (TULAREMIA)

Inoculation

- ulcerating papule develops at site of inoculation followed by abrupt onset of fever, malaise, fatigue

Transmission

- blood-sucking arthropods
- deer flies and ticks (wood and dog) contaminate bite with feces
- ingestion of contaminated meat or H_2O
- handling infected tissues; inhalation; bites from infected animals

Diagnosis

- specimens
- isolation
  - ⇒ cysteine–glucose–blood agar
- id/serology

Treatment

- streptomycin
- vaccination

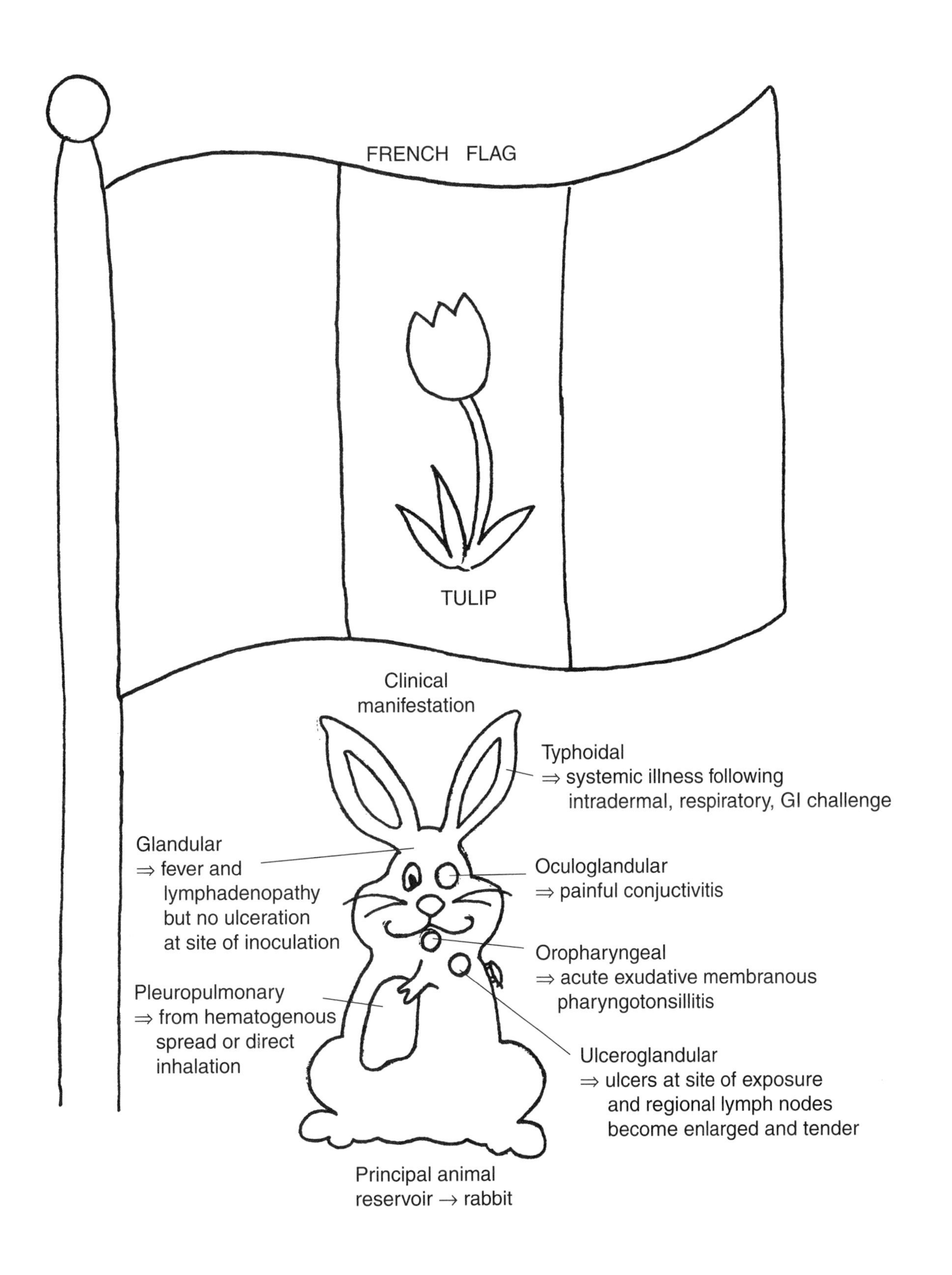
FRENCH FLAG
TULIP
Clinical manifestation
Typhoidal ⇒ systemic illness following intradermal, respiratory, GI challenge
Glandular ⇒ fever and lymphadenopathy but no ulceration at site of inoculation
Oculoglandular ⇒ painful conjuctivitis
Oropharyngeal ⇒ acute exudative membranous pharyngotonsillitis
Pleuropulmonary ⇒ from hematogenous spread or direct inhalation
Ulceroglandular ⇒ ulcers at site of exposure and regional lymph nodes become enlarged and tender
Principal animal reservoir → rabbit

NOTES

Four Species

P. multocida—primary pathogen in humans
P. haemolytica
P. pneumotropica, and
P. ureae—less common pathogen
P. multocida—(**multi**vitamins)
P. haemolytica—(heme)
P. pneumotropica—(pneumonia fighters)
P. ureae—(urea)

Reservoirs

- domestic and wild animals
  - ⇒ cat, dog, swine

Transmission: (3 ways)

- animal bites and scratches (most common)
- non-bite animal exposure
- no known animal exposure
  - ⇒ patients with upper respiratory infection

Pathogenesis (3 ways)

- soft tissue infection
- chronic respiratory tract infection
- systemic infections
  - ⇒ bloodstream invasion (hemorrhagic septicemia)
  - ⇒ tissues infected (meninges, brain, liver, joints)
  - ⇒ fatal infection uncommon

Diagnosis

- clinical manifestation
  - ⇒ cellulitis within 24 hrs of bite wound or cat scratch

Treatment

- ampicillin
- recovery slow

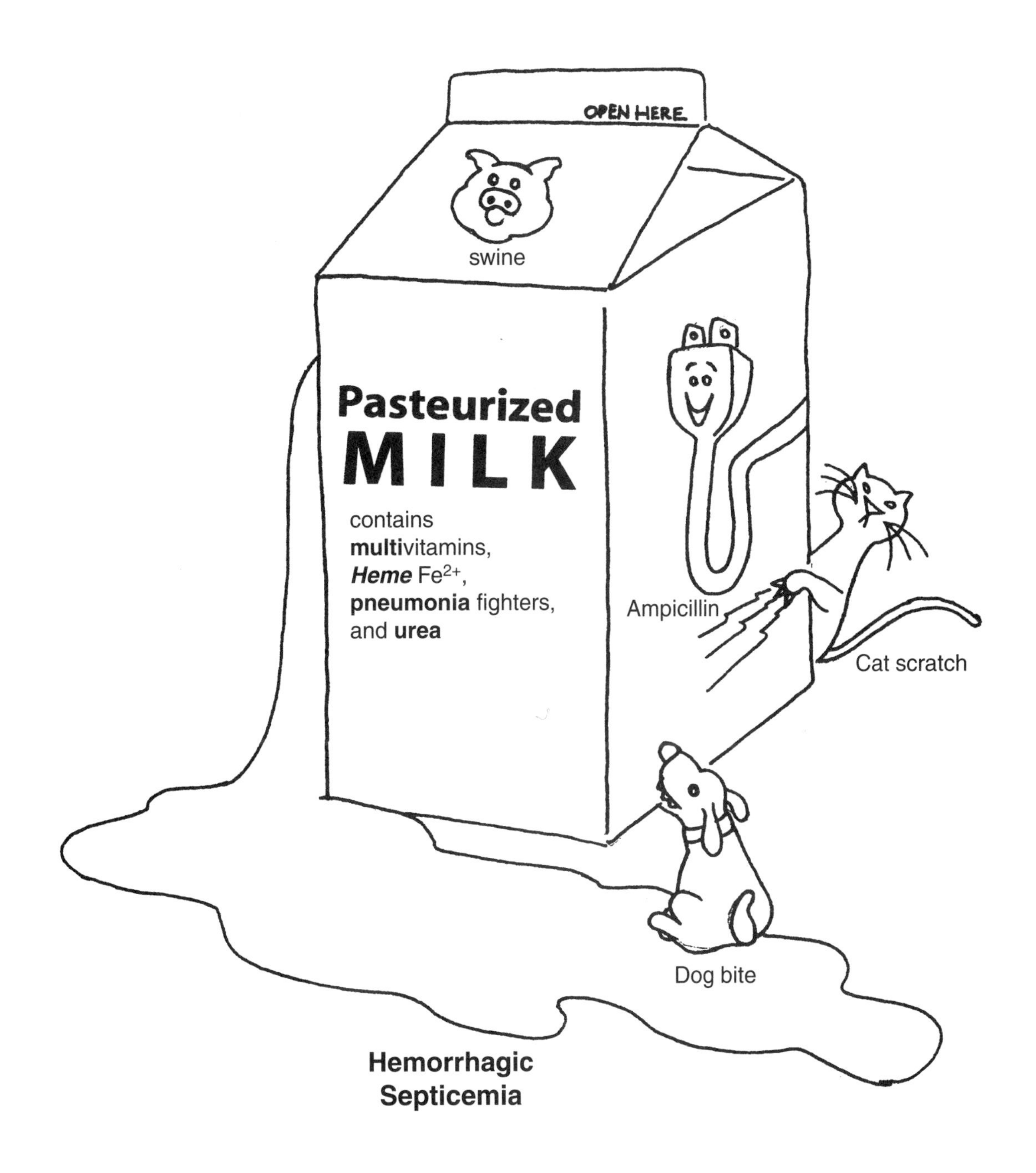
OPEN HERE
swine
Pasteurized
MILK
contains
multivitamins,
Heme Fe2+,
pneumonia fighters,
and urea
Ampicillin
Cat scratch
Dog bite
Hemorrhagic
Septicemia

NOTES

- ⇒ border of basketball backboard
- small gram-negative bacillus
- 3 species
  - ⇒ *B. pertussis*→whooping cough
    - ⇒ pretty Tess
    - ⇒ "hooping cough"
  - ⇒ *B. parapertussis*→mild with cough
  - ⇒ *B. bronchiseptica*→animal pathogen of upper respiratory tract
- *B. pertussis* requires complex growth medium
  - ⇒ Bordet-Gengou medium (potato, blood and glycerol)

Transmission

- highly contagious disease spread by upper respiratory secretions
- naturally acquired *B. pertussis* infection only occurs in humans
- old and young susceptible
- cell-mediated immunity important
- Antigenic/virulence factors (A–E)
  - A) capsule-only *B. pertussis*
  - B) tracheal cytotoxin
    - ⇒ part of *B. pertussis,* cell wall
    - ⇒ interferes with and dislodges ciliated epithelial cells along the trachea
  - C) pertussis toxin
    - ⇒ severe cough
  - D) filamentous hemagglutinin
    - ⇒ mediates attachment
  - E) adenylate cyclase toxin ATP→cAMP

Pathogenesis (1–6)

1) incubation
   - attaches and noninvasive
2) catarrhal, prodromal, preparoxysmal stage
   - patient develops non-specific upper respiratory symptoms
   - **patient most infectious**
3) paroxysmal, spasmodic stage
   - lower respiratory involved
   - severe cough
4) convalescent stage
   - decreased cough severity
5) complications
   - 2° bacterial infection—otitis media, pneumonia
   - seizures and encephalopathy
6) immunity
   - lasts 15–20 years

Treatment

- erythromycin
  - ⇒ "This is EERY!"
- vaccination
  - ⇒ original and acellular
    - ⇒ ACEL-IMUNE

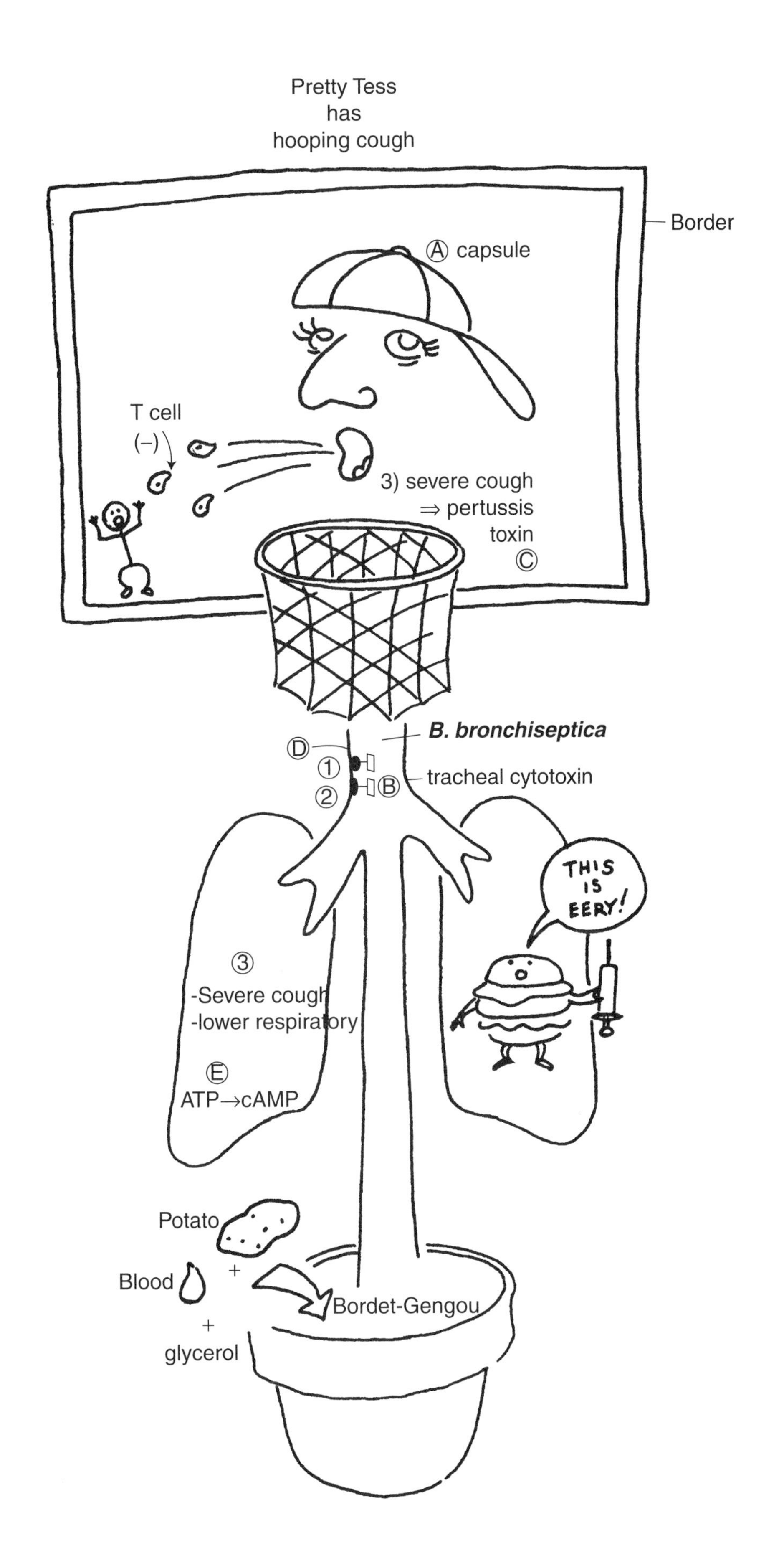
Pretty Tess
has
hooping cough
Border
Ⓐ capsule
T cell
(–)
3) severe cough
⇒ pertussis
toxin
Ⓒ
B. bronchiseptica
Ⓓ
①
②
Ⓑ
tracheal cytotoxin
THIS
IS
EERY!
③
-Severe cough
-lower respiratory
Ⓔ
ATP→cAMP
Potato
Blood
+
+
glycerol
Bordet-Gengou

NOTES

BRUCELLA

⇒ Bruce Springsteen's guitar

brucellosis—acute febrile disease or a chronic disease of widely varying symptomatology

⇒ six species of importance:

B. melitensis—goats and sheep
B. abortus—cattle
B. suis—swine
B. canis—dogs
B. ovis—sheep
B. neotomae—rodents

Synonyms

undulant fever, Rio Grande fever, goat fever, Bang's disease (*B. abortus* infection in cattle)

Morphology

- small gram-negative bacilli
- non-motile
- non-spore-forming

Physiology

- enriched media required for isolation
- *brucella* use **erythritol**
  - ⇒ present in placenta of many animals but not humans
- viscerotropin
  - ⇒ *Brucella* frequently colonizes placenta of animals resulting in abortion

Transmission

- skin inoculation
- ingestion—unpasteurized milk or uncooked infected meat
- inhalation
- conjunctiva inoculation
- laboratory acquired
- person-to-person (rare)

Incidence

- occupational exposure
  - ⇒ most cases seen in slaughterhouse workers, livestock handlers, and vets
  - ⇒ mostly in rural areas

Antigenic/virulence factors

- A and M antigens—all *Brucella* have them but in different proportions
- lipopolysaccharide
  - ⇒ sensitivity of host to endotoxin plays a role in pathogenicity
- capsule

Pathogenesis

1) from portal of entry→ingested in PMNs→intracellular multiplication→ *Brucella* carried to lymph nodes→ bloodstream→organ invasion (especially RE system: liver, spleen, bone marrow, lymphatic system)→small granulomatous lesions are formed

Clinical Manifestations

- asymptomatic brucellosis
- acute: fever only symptom
- relapsing: gradual step-by-step increase, then decrease of temperature→occurring several times
- localized in organs
  - ⇒ pulmonary, bones/joints (most common), genitourinary tract, CNS (blurred vision), cardiovascular
- Strain 19 disease
  - ⇒ *B. abortus*→cattle
  - ⇒ vets have most often

- convalescence—long 1–4 months
- immunity—not absolute

Diagnosis

- isolation and identification
- growth in basic fuchsin and thionine
- production of H_2S
- urease hydrolysis
- agglutination

Treatment

- doxycycline + aminoglycoside

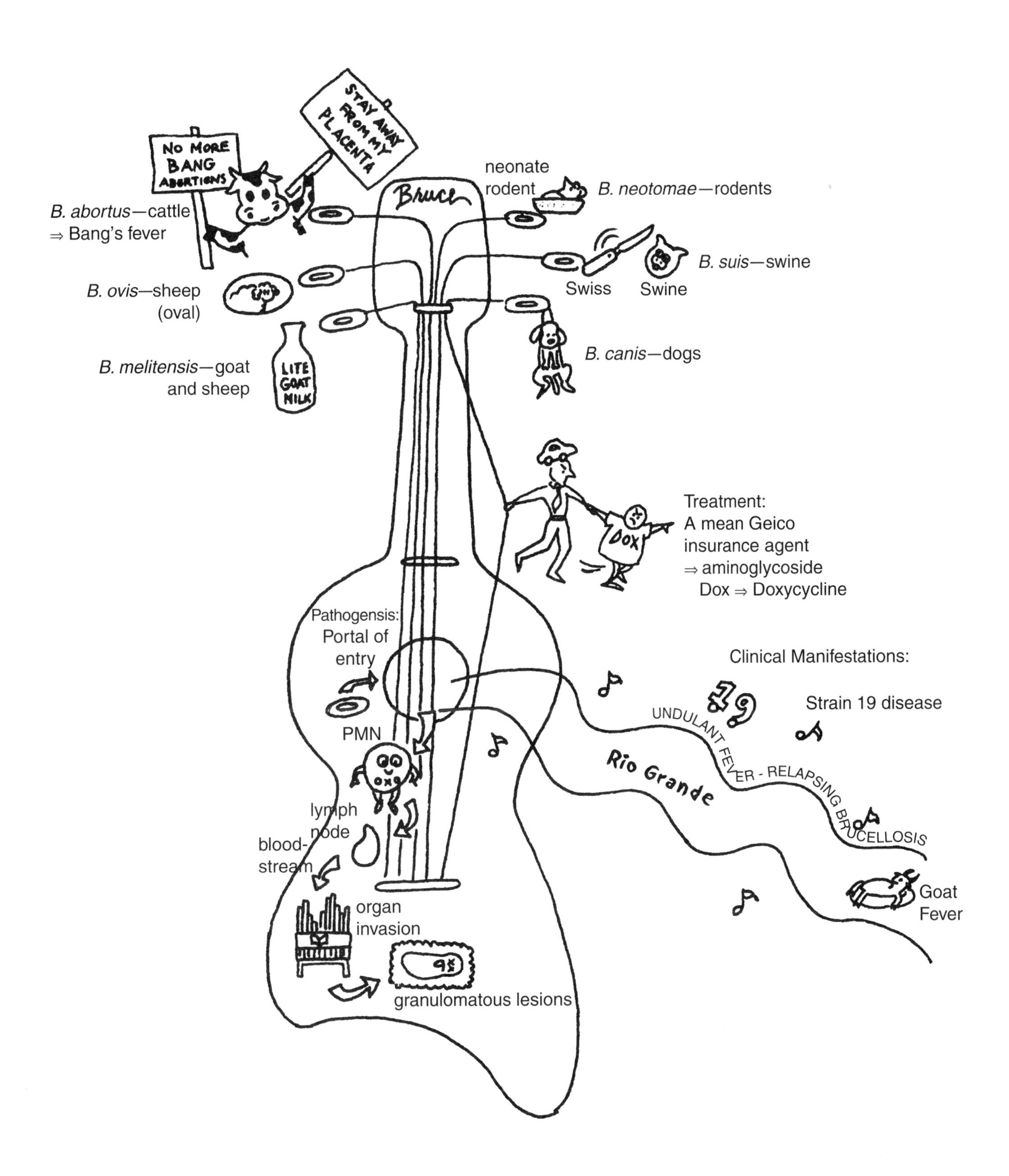
STAY AWAY FROM MY PLACENTA
NO MORE BANG ABORTIONS
Bruce
neonate rodent
B. neotomae—rodents
B. abortus—cattle
⇒ Bang's fever
Swiss
Swine
B. suis—swine
B. ovis—sheep
(oval)
B. canis—dogs
B. melitensis—goat
and sheep
LITE GOAT MILK
Treatment:
A mean Geico
insurance agent
⇒ aminoglycoside
Dox ⇒ Doxycycline
DOX
Pathogensis:
Portal of
entry
PMN
lymph
node
blood-
stream
organ
invasion
granulomatous lesions
Clinical Manifestations:
19
Strain 19 disease
UNDULANT FEVER - RELAPSING BRUCELLOSIS
Rio Grande
Goat
Fever

Mycobacteria

NOTES

General

- cause chronic lung infections (TB)
- disseminated infection (leprosy)
- grow very slowly⇒cane
- *M. tuberculosis*⇒My co. tubular
  - ⇒ **simple growth requirements**—trace metals **asparagine** and glycerol
  - ⇒ "asparagus" "glistening bubble"
- **mycobacterial acid-fast stain**⇒upside down acid jar
  - ⇒ **retain dye (carbolfuchsin) following discoloration with acidic alcohol**

Test difference

***Mycobacterium*—resist decolorization with acidic ethanol whereas corynebacteria and *Nocardia* resist mineral acids**

M. leprae

- cannot be cultivated in vitro but *M. tuberculosis* can
- Mitsuda skin test
  - ⇒ not for diagnosis but for determining patient on immunity spectrum
- causes granulomatous lesions
- organisms in lesions are intracellular and proliferate in macrophages
- chronic slow progress; mutilating and disfiguring lesions
- predilection for skin and for nerve
  cutaneous—lepromas
  neuronal—anesthesia of peripheral nerves
- 3 phases of disease
  1) lepromatous—progressive; lepra cells (foamy macrophages); lepromin test ⊖; prognosis poor
  2) tuberculoid: healing; test ⊕
  3) intermediate—bacteria in necrotic areas; prognosis fair; test ⊕
- treatment with dapsone (diaminodiphenyl sulfone)
  - ⇒ diamonds of cat ears
- diagnosis with scrapings
  - ⇒ ⊕ for acid-fast bacilli
- **not highly contagious:** transmitted through lesion contact with open abrasion
- genetic factors (HLA)—predispose

Mycobacterium tuberculosis

- tubercle bacilli
- strains differ—grow in rods or as aggregated long arrangements→serpentine cords
  - ⇒ (serpents)
- walls contain peptidoglycan with diaminopimelate
  - ⇒ high lipid content⇒peptidoglycan (Pepsi)
  - ⇒ diaminopimelate (diamonds ◊)
- obligate aerobe—"loves oxygen"
- in ordinary synthetic liquid media grow in adherent clumps→surface pellicle
- nutritional preference for lipids (egg yolks)
- inhibited by long chain FA (high concentration) stimulated at low concentration

Virulence

- virulent strains grow on liquid surface or solid as intertwining serpentine cords
  - ⇒ aggregate with long axes parallel
  - ⇒ cords→correlated with surface lipid→cord factor

Lipids

- high lipid content (60% dry wt)
- lipid-rich cell wall
  - ⇒ impermeable to stains; acid-fastness; resistance to acid/alkali; resistance to antibody and complement
- mycolic acids
- cord factor: extraction renders nonvirulent strain
  - ⇒ inhibits PMNs; essential for virulence and serpentine cords
- *wax D*: mycolic acid and glycopeptide; ↑ immunogenicity⇒"ear wax D"
- sulfatides: potentiate toxicity of cord factor; promote survival in macrophages by preventing phagolysosome formation
  - ⇒ "sulfur tide"

Pathogenesis

inhalation→self-limiting lesion→1° infection →non-specific pneumonitis in well-aerated peripheral zone→DT hypersensitivity→ granulomatous inflammation→tubercles (small lumps containing phagocytic cells)→(bacilli also carried to lymph nodes→body) caseation necrosis→scar formation→
Ghon complex→healed 1° complex lesion
  - ⇒ "Gandhi is complexed"

- reactivation disease: reactivation of long-dormant foci remaining from 1° infection (in genitourinary tract, bones/joints, lymph nodes, pleura, and peritoneum)
- disseminated TB (miliary)→rupture of caseous lesion into pulmonary vein
- resistance varies with race
  - ⇒ ↑ in Indians, Eskimos, and blacks
  - ⇒ malnutrition (↓ protein), overcrowding, and stress ↓ resistance to disease
- Antibodies no role in immunity with *M. tuberculosis*
- Koch phenomenon—↑ attack of 2° infection
- *M. Tuberculosis* niacin positive→nice on t-shirt
- enhanced macrophage activity is nonspecific
  - ⇒ macrophages will kill all other bacteria at accelerated rate, but only *M. tuberculosis* antigen will activate them

Diagnosis

acid-fast bacilli in smears→culture

Tuberculin Test

DTH (delayed type hypersensitivity)→past infection if ⊕, but not necessarily active infection

Treatment

Rifampin + isoniazid is the best; streptomycin is ototoxic

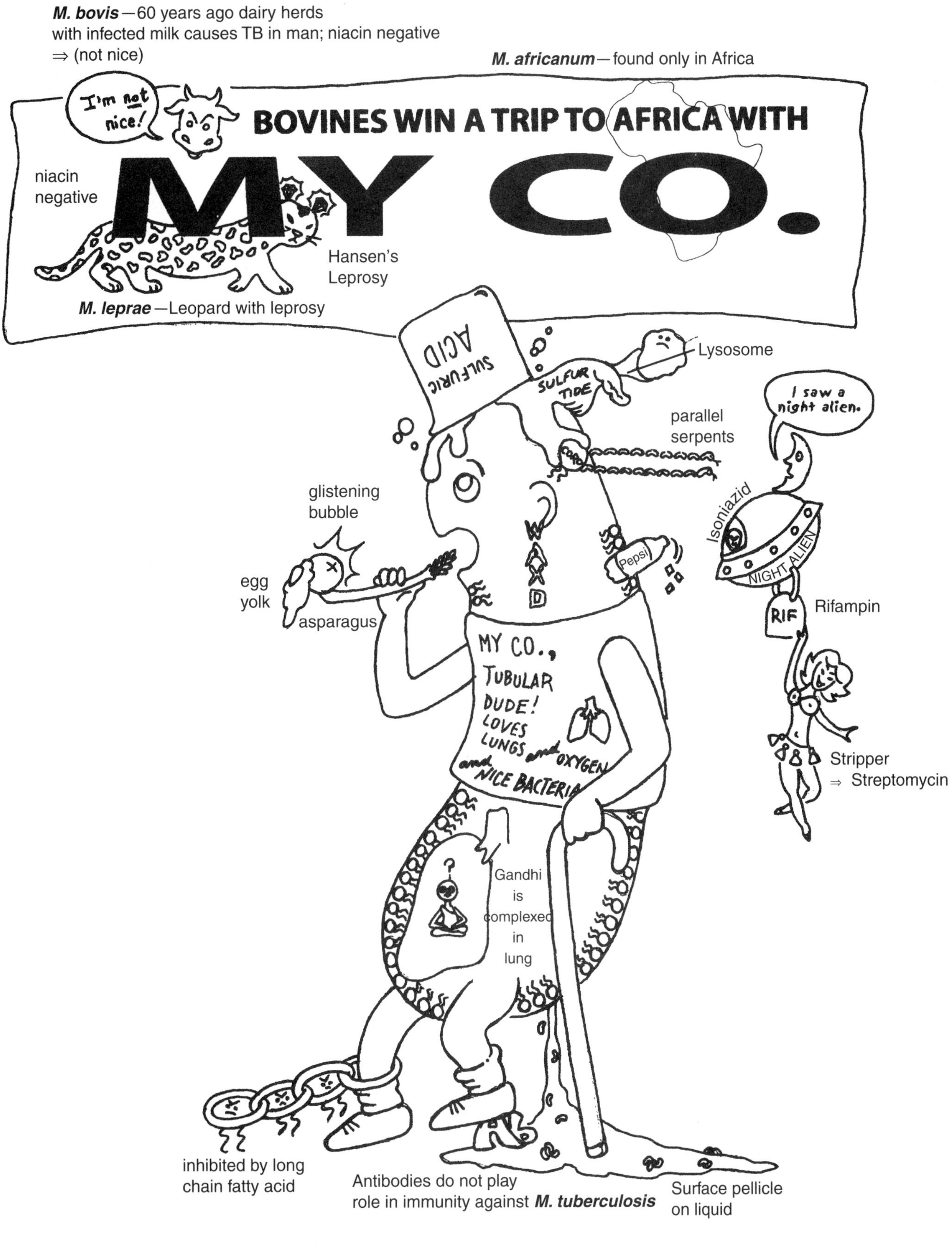

M. bovis — 60 years ago dairy herds with infected milk causes TB in man; niacin negative ⇒ (not nice)

M. africanum — found only in Africa

I'm not nice!

BOVINES WIN A TRIP TO AFRICA WITH

MY CO.

niacin negative

Hansen's Leprosy

M. leprae — Leopard with leprosy

SULFURIC ACID

Lysosome

SULFUR TIDE

I saw a night alien.

parallel serpents

CORD

glistening bubble

Isoniazid

NIGHT ALIEN

WAX D

Pepsi

egg yolk

asparagus

RIF

Rifampin

MY CO., TUBULAR DUDE! LOVES LUNGS and OXYGEN and NICE BACTERIA

Stripper ⇒ Streptomycin

Gandhi is complexed in lung

inhibited by long chain fatty acid

Antibodies do not play role in immunity against ***M. tuberculosis***

Surface pellicle on liquid

NOTES

⇒ My cop gives plasma

LEGIONELLA PNEUMOPHILA

- **causes "Legionnaire's disease"**
- **short rods**
- stains poorly, may be gram-negative
- stains better with **silver stains**
- all species have a single common **flagellar antigen**
- most clinical disease caused by *L. pneumophila* serogroup 1
- **intracellular parasite; phagocytosed by both PMN and macrophages**
- grows intracellularly
- antibody **enhances phago**cytosis but not killing
- activated macrophages do kill bacteria (**cell mediated immunity** important)
- **produce cytotoxin→inhibits PMN oxidative metabolism**
- occasionally **dust-borne** but usually traced to H_2O cooling towers connected to air conditioning (aerosols); person-to-person infection rare
- **2 diseases** caused by *L. pneumophila*
  1. **Pneumonia (L. disease)**
  2. **Pontiac fever (self-limiting with fever, chills, headache, myalgia)**
- majority of cases occurs in summers ♂ 2 : ♂ 1; >50 years old
- organism usually found in lung but may spread with dissemination occurring in immunosuppressed patients; **sudden onset with fever, chills, myalgia, and dry cough**→may progress to severe pneumonia
- **organisms produce B-lactamase**
  Two important species
  (1) ***L. micdadei*—Pittsburgh** pneumonia agent; different from *L. pneumophila* in DNA;⇒macadamian nuts
  (2) *L. bozemanii*—differ in DNA from *L. pneumophila*⇒Bose radio

Diagnosis

fluorescent antibody stain; lung culture

Treatment

erythromycin, rifampin

L-FORMS

- **variants of certain bacteria that can arise spontaneously** and can replicate in the form of small filterable elements with absent cell walls
- **capable of reversion** back to parent strain
- **agents** that convert parent to L-form—**antibiotics, LiCl, caffeine, lysozyme, specific antibody plus complement**
- highly susceptible to osmotic pressure and need stabilizing agents: *salt, sugars, polypeptides, and spermines*

MYCOPLASMA

- **primary atypical pneumonia** *(PAP)* caused by Mycoplasma
- **smallest known free-living organism**
- extremely pleomorphic because no cell wall
- stain poorly—not gram stainable
- **on solid media form minute colonies with fried egg appearance**
- **require rich growth medium** (serum protein and sterol)
- **susceptible to kanamycin, tetracycline, gold salts, but not thallium acetate→ resistant to sulfonamides and penicillin; more susceptible to killing by H_2O, saline, and soap**
- ***M. hominis* and T strains** (*Ureaplasma urealyticus*)
  - ⇒ **T strains require urea for growth→ produce urease**
  - ⇒ **M. hominin causes genitourinary infections**
- **PAP—Caused by *M. pneumoniae***
- **Eaton's agent** differs from all other human Mycoplasma
- tissue strains more virulent than agar-grown strains
- cold agglutinins, *streptococcus* MG agglutinins, and **growth inhibiting antibodies in mycoplasma infections**
- **diagnosis** by CF test (lipid-antigen complex) or immfluorescence
- **treatment with tetracycline or kanamycin; immunity—due to magnitude of serum antibody against organism**
- **DTH reaction—correlates with severity of disease**

Treatment

Kanamycin⇒Kansas
tetracycline⇒tetracycle
gold salts⇒gold saw

Resistant to

Penicillin⇒penny
Sulfonamides⇒magician on sulfur
Other illustration explanations:
Sterol and protein⇒steer
T-strain⇒tete
Urease and genitourinary infections⇒urine
M. pneumoniae cause PAP⇒Lungs with PAP

PROTOPLASTS AND SPHEROPLASTS

- **formed by cell-wall degrading enzymes**
- morphologically equivalent to L-forms but **L-form restricted to cells that can multiply**; protoplasts and spheroplasts restricted to cells that don't replicate

protoplast—gram-positive cell with no remnants of cell wall left

spheroplast—gram-negative cell that contains remnants of cell wall

Mycoplasmas (PPO, PPLO), L-Forms, and *Legionella Pneumophila* (Wall-Less Bacteria)

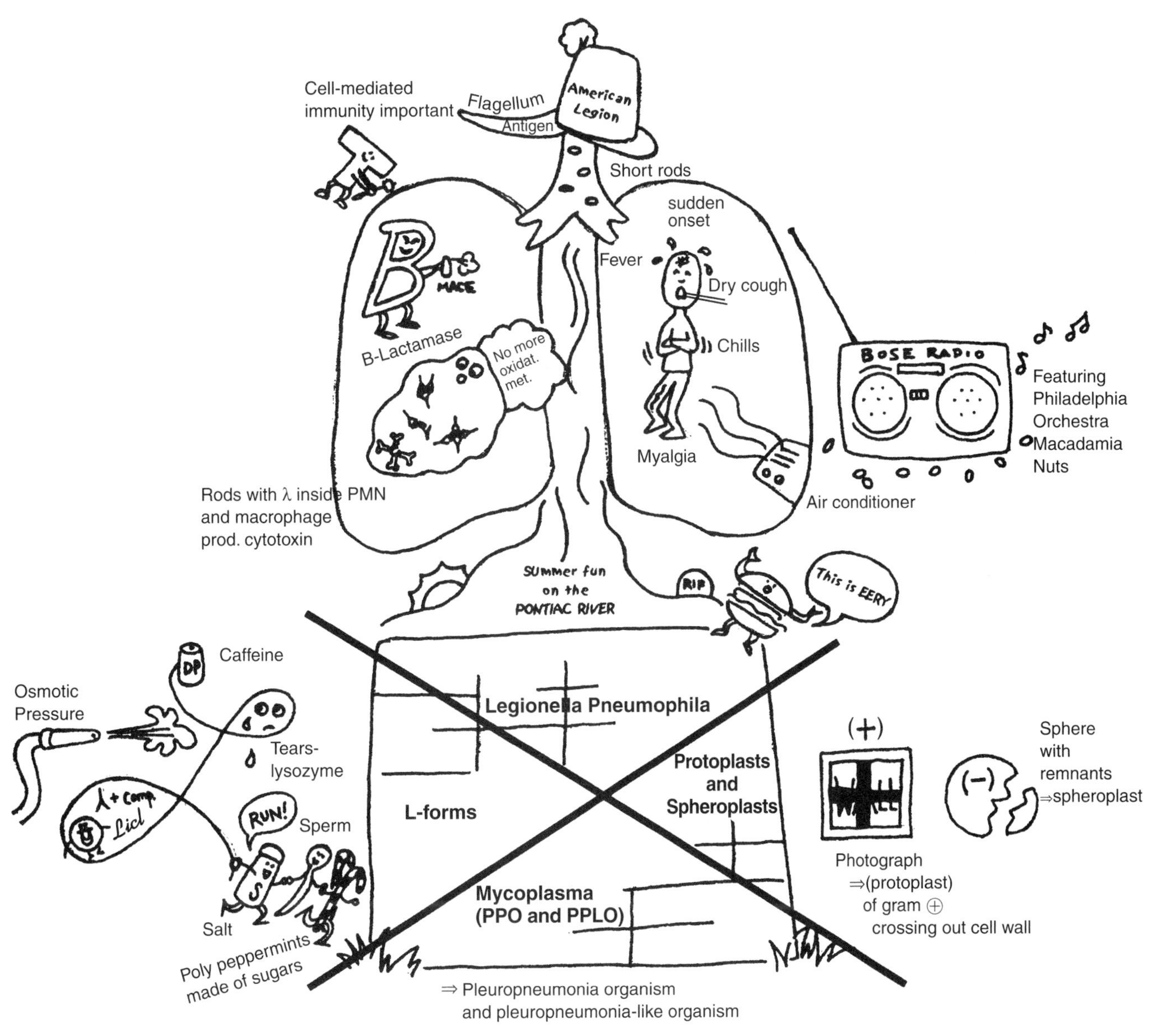

"My cop gives plasma, which takes the shape of its container!"

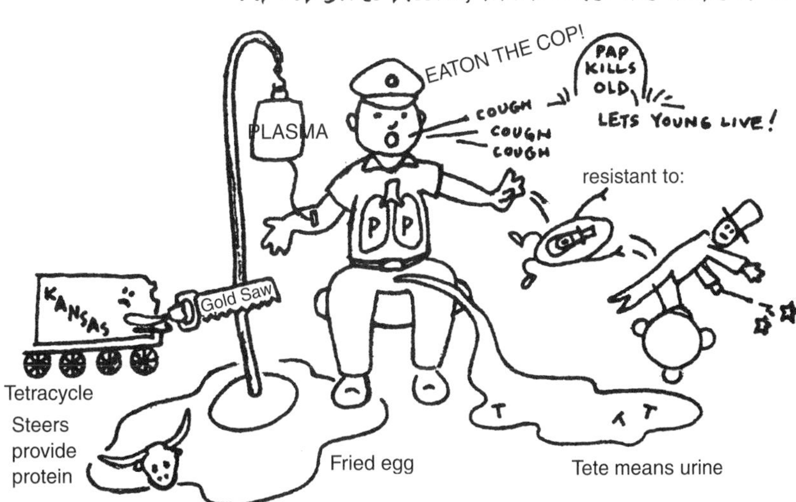

RICKETTSIA

- most **rickettsias are conveyed by arthropod vectors but *Coxiella burnetii* transmitted by inhalation of contaminated dust**
- **multiply in vascular endothelial cells→** with local pathology (vasculitis and thrombosis) distributed through body: CNS, skin (rash), heart, lungs, kidney
- **small pleomorphic coccobacilli**
- **obligate intracellular parasites**
- contain **DNA, RNA; divide by binary fission; cell-wall (gram-negative)**

NOTES

- **susceptible to tetracycline and chloramphenicol**
  ⇒ tetracycle ⇒colorful fin
- 4 genera: **Rickettsia, Rochalimaea, Coxiella, Ehrlichia**

TYPHUS FEVER GROUP

⇒ wears tie

epidemic louse-borne typhus (*R. prowazekii*)

- **humans only reservoir**
- **louse dies of infection**
- *R. prowazekii* multiplies in gut of louse→ louse feeds→then transmitted
- symptoms: fever, headache, myalgia
- **rash appears on 4th day**
  ⇒ **first on trunk then limbs but not face**
- maculopapular rash with petechia
- **CNS involvement; uremia**
- severe illness
- **Brills disease**→recrudescence
  ⇒ *grill*

endemic flea-borne murine typhus (*R. typhi*)

⇒ (marine)

- not fatal in rats or fleas
- **humans accidental host when flea bitten**
- person-to-person transmission does not occur
- similar to louse typhus but less severe

SPOTTED FEVER GROUP

⇒ have spots

Rocky Mountain spotted fever (*R. rickettsii*)—

⇒ Rick

- **rodents/dogs reservoirs**
  ⇒ their ticks bite humans
- **transvarial transmission tick is both reservoir and vector**
- incubation—7 days
- headache, fever, myalgia
- **rash first on hands/feet then trunk and face**
- rash
  ⇒ maculopapular with petechia
- **death due to circulatory collapse and kidney failure**

boutonneuse fever⇒boutonniere
(*R. conorii*)⇒conroy

⇒ Mediterranean fever or tickbite fever occurring in Africa and India
⇒ resembles Rocky Mountain but milder

rickettsial pox⇒Ricket pal
(R. a.k.a. rii)⇒a.k.a. rii

- US and Russia
- mild illness—vesicular rash and eschar at the site of the bite
- all have common complement-fixing antigen

SCRUB TYPHUS

⇒ wearing surgical mask

scrub typhus (*R. tsutsugamushi*)

⇒ wearing tutu

- chiefly seen in India, SE Asia, and Australia
- transmitted by mites (trombiculid); mites are chiggers
- humans accidental host
- eschar at bite site

TRENCH FEVER

⇒ in a trench

(*Rochalimaea quintana*)

now *Bartonella quintana*⇒5 barmaids named Ella

- **transmitted by body louse**⇒"every BODY's favorite louse"
- rash resembles that seen in typhoid fever
- **course is short (5 days)**

***can be cultivated on blood agar under 10% CO_2 (differs from all others in this)**

Q FEVER

⇒ letter q

Coxiella burnetii

⇒ Carol Burnett

- **natural cycle maintained by tick**
  ⇒ *C. burnetii*—excreted in cow/sheep milk, urine, feces, and placentas
- is inhaled or ingested in unpasteurized milk

***no rash observed**

HUMAN GRANULOCYTIC EHRLICHIOSIS (HGE)

⇒ *Ehrlichia canis*
⇒ "licking canine"

- recent
- fatalities frequent
- death associated with **monocytic ehrlichiosis→2° to organ failure**

Treatment

with chloramphenicol and tetracycline

TREATMENT, PROPHYLAXIS, DIAGNOSIS

Treatment

tetracycline (tetracycle) and chloramphenicol (colored fin)

Prophylaxis

- vector control
- mass application of insecticides for human lice
- elimination of rats for rat fleas
- vaccines→formalin-inactivated

Diagnosis

- blood agar under 10% CO_2 for *Rochalimaea*
- **stain poorly but are gram-negative**
- indirect fluorescent antibody test
- complement-fixation tests
- **Weil-Felix test**—agglutination of *Proteus vulgaris* strains Ox-19

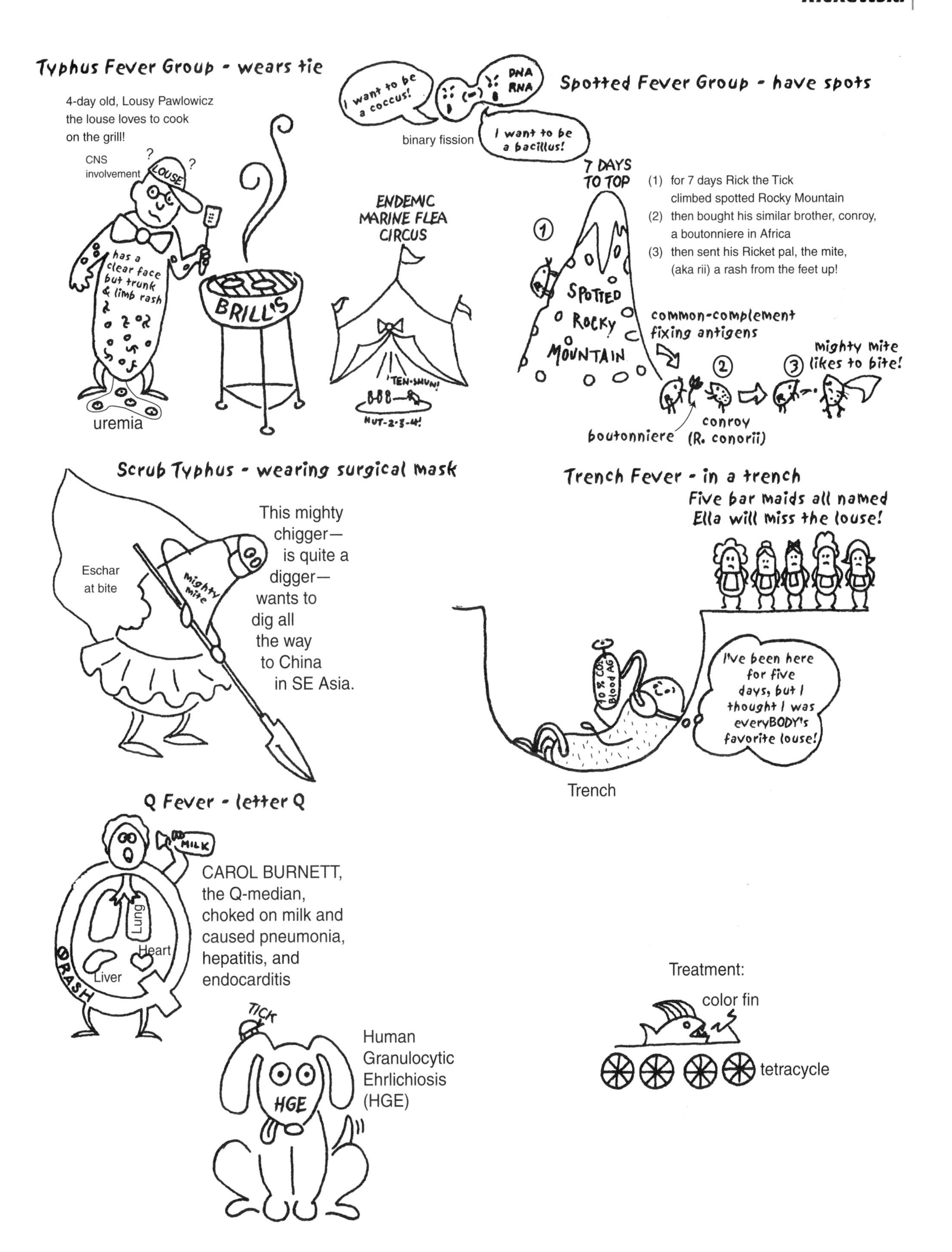
Typhus Fever Group - wears tie
4-day old, Lousy Pawlowicz
the louse loves to cook
on the grill!
CNS
involvement
LOUSE
has a
clear face
but trunk
& limb rash
uremia
BRILL'S
ENDEMIC
MARINE FLEA
CIRCUS
'TEN-SHUN!
HUT-2-3-4!
I want to be
a coccus!
DNA
RNA
I want to be
a bacillus!
binary fission
Spotted Fever Group - have spots
7 DAYS
TO TOP
(1) for 7 days Rick the Tick
climbed spotted Rocky Mountain
(2) then bought his similar brother, conroy,
a boutonniere in Africa
(3) then sent his Ricket pal, the mite,
(aka rii) a rash from the feet up!
SPOTTED
ROCKY
MOUNTAIN
common-complement
fixing antigens
mighty mite
likes to bite!
boutonniere
conroy
(R. conorii)
Scrub Typhus - wearing surgical mask
Eschar
at bite
mighty
mite
This mighty
chigger—
is quite a
digger—
wants to
dig all
the way
to China
in SE Asia.
Trench Fever - in a trench
Five bar maids all named
Ella will miss the louse!
10 % CO2
Blood AG
I've been here
for five
days, but I
thought I was
everyBODY's
favorite louse!
Trench
Q Fever - letter Q
MILK
CAROL BURNETT,
the Q-median,
choked on milk and
caused pneumonia,
hepatitis, and
endocarditis
Lung
Heart
Liver
RASH
TICK
HGE
Human
Granulocytic
Ehrlichiosis
(HGE)
Treatment:
color fin
tetracycle

NOTES

CHLAMYDIAE

⇒ clam

- obligate **intracellular parasites:**
  - ⇒ predilection for columnar epithelial cells lining mucous membranes
- lack energy-producing enzyme systems
- contain both **DNA and RNA**: possess ribosomes; divide by **binary fission**, have **cell wall** containing **peptidoglycan; ferment glucose liberating CO_2; sensitive to tetracycline and sulfonamides**
- groups: *C. trachomatis, C. psittaci, C. pneumoniae*
- infectious particle is called an **elementary body** that is a coccoid form about .3 µm in diameter→enlarges to form reticulate body **(initial body)→divides** by binary fission to form more **reticulate bodies**, and **from these**→numerous small **elementary bodies** develop
- multiplication takes place within **cytoplasmic vacuole** in host cell→ **Chlamydiae being embedded in a matrix to comprise a colony is the pathognomonic inclusion**
  - ⇒ **matrix of *C. trachomatis* stains with iodine—*C. psittaci* does not** (white)
  - ⇒ **inclusion of *C. trachomatis* is compact—*C. psittaci* is diffuse→pale**
  - ⇒ **inclusion of *C. pneumoniae* is pear-shaped, diffuse, and does not stain with iodine**
- **genome is circular DNA**
- staining—resemble gram-negative but don't stain well with Gram stain
- **Giemsa stain** and iodine for matrix of those that stain with it (*C. trachomatis*)
- antigens—**family-specific antigen** (glycolipid); **type-specific antigen** (a protein)→in cell wall against which protective Abs are formed
- cell penetration→elementary bodies attach to host cell (are phagocytosed)→ enhanced by centrifugation of elementary bodies onto cell treated with cycloheximide (arrests nucleic acid synthesis)

C. TRACHOMATIS

Diseases caused by *C. trachomatis:* **trachoma, inclusion conjunctivitis,** (⇒ TRIC agent's) **nonspecific urethritis, cervicitis, salpingitis, neonatal pneumonitis, lymphogranuloma venereum**

- **trachoma**—disease of conjunctiva and cornea; **cause of blindness**; transmission is from eye to eye (fingers, flies); organism causes inflammation of the conjunctiva of the upper part of the eye; infiltration by lymphocytes and plasma cells→**pannus develops**; scarring of upper eyelid→ inversion of lid margin (entropin)→with damage to cornea by eyelashes (trichiasis; →corneal inflammation→blindness

Treatment

- **early with tetracycline or sulfonamides**
- **inclusion conjunctivitis**—genital infection of one person conveyed to the eye of another→newborn→developing **inclusion blennorrhea** (not subject to eradication with silver nitrate)→severe purulent conjunctivitis develops during the first 2 weeks of life
  - ⇒ **swimming pool conjunctivitis**→ adults and older children usually contract the ocular disease through infection via genital secretions in poorly chlorinated swimming pools
  - ⇒ infection primarily affects the conjunctiva of the lower eyelid with lymphoid follicle formation but without serious scarring
- genital infection: genital infection transmitted venereally→nonspecific urethritis (*C. trachomatis*)→can cause cervicitis and salpingitis; pneumonia of infants—first few months of life; fever absent
- lymphogranuloma venereum (LGV)→ serotypes (L1, L2, L3); venereally transmitted; small initial papule→ inflammation of lymph nodes with suppuration **(bubo)**; sinus formation; can involve rectum (proctitis)→renal stricture

Diagnosis

observation of inclusion in scrapings; Giemsa with iodine; isolation of *Chlamydia* in yolk sac of chick embryo; Frei test of LGV ⇒ intradermal inoculation of *Chlamydia* antigen grown in chick embryo→detects any *Chlamydia* infection not specific for LGV

C. PSITTACI

⇒ Polly **sits** 1° pneumonia⇒lungs

- psittacosis—ornithosis is a zoonosis acquired by humans from psittacine **(parrot-like) birds**; birds develop chronic carrier state; organism excreted in feces; in humans→presents as 1° atypical pneumonia→treatment with tetracycline; person-to-person transmission (by aerosol)→notably in hospitals

C. PNEUMONIAE

First called TWAR (***Ta****iwan* ***A****cute* ***R****espiratory* Illness)

- cause relatively mild upper respiratory tract infection; occasionally pneumonia can develop; may require hospitalization; sore throat, low grade fever, and persistent cough are common symptoms; transmitted human to human; sensitive to erythromycin and tetracycline

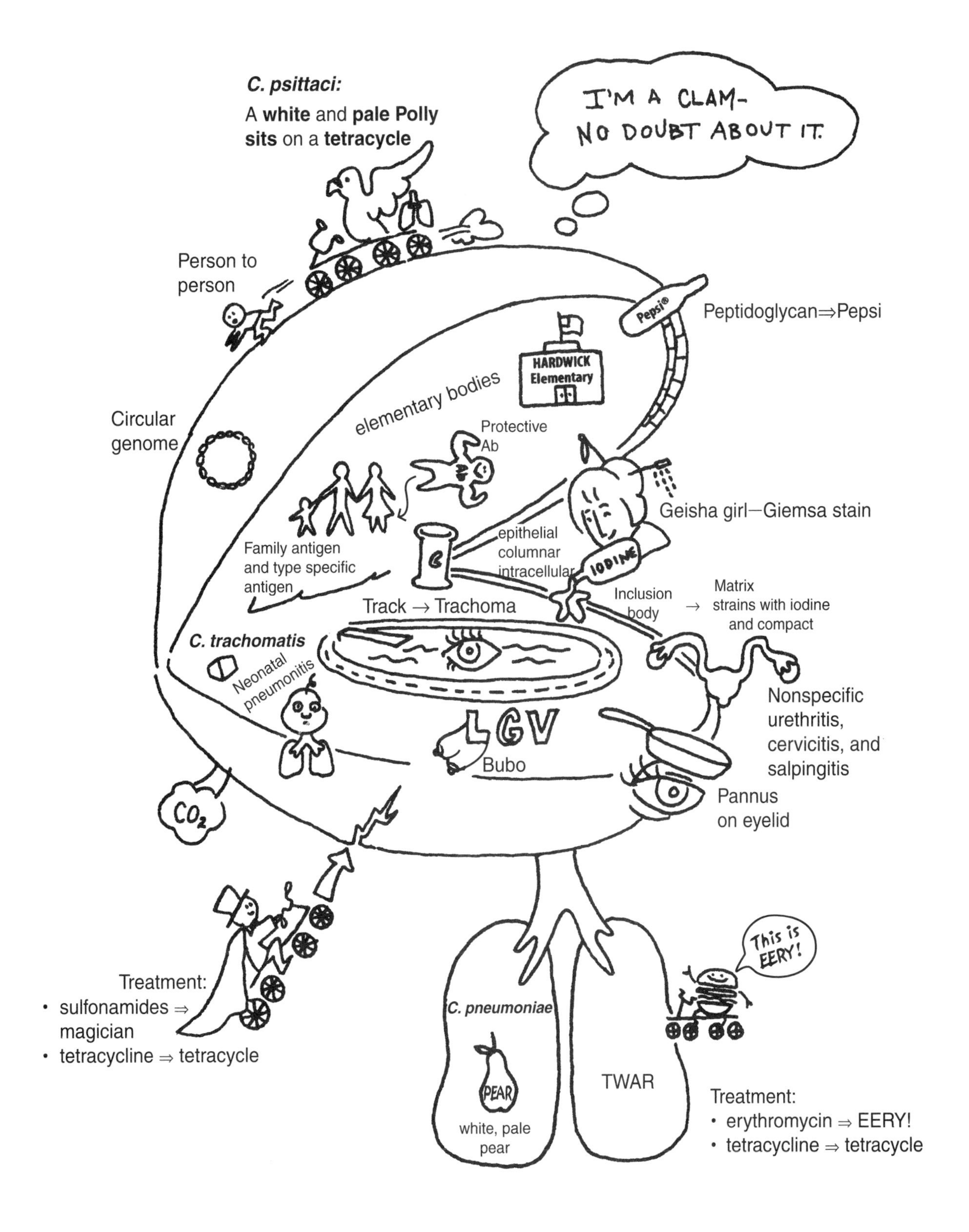
C. psittaci:
A white and pale Polly sits on a tetracycle
I'M A CLAM- NO DOUBT ABOUT IT.
Person to person
Pepsi®
Peptidoglycan⇒Pepsi
HARDWICK Elementary
elementary bodies
Circular genome
Protective Ab
Geisha girl—Giemsa stain
Family antigen and type specific antigen
epithelial columnar intracellular
IODINE
Inclusion body → Matrix strains with iodine and compact
Track → Trachoma
C. trachomatis
Neonatal pneumonitis
Nonspecific urethritis, cervicitis, and salpingitis
LGV
Bubo
Pannus on eyelid
CO_2
Treatment:
• sulfonamides ⇒ magician
• tetracycline ⇒ tetracycle
This is EERY!
C. pneumoniae
PEAR
white, pale pear
TWAR
Treatment:
• erythromycin ⇒ EERY!
• tetracycline ⇒ tetracycle

NOTES

all share characteristics of

- gram-negative; non-spore-forming obligate aerobe or falcultative anaeraose

Bartonella bacilliformis

- *Bartonella*⇒Barton Eilla (Carrion's disease⇒carries disease)
- (Carrion's disease) occurs in Andean valleys of Colombia, Equador, and Peru; transmission by sand fly; bacteremia initial phase; RBC lysed; nodular lesions form; death from severe anemia; diagnosis by blood films and by isolation of organism

***Calymmatobacterium granulomatis* (donovanosis)**

- tropical climates; transmission by sex or autoinoculation
- clinical; granuloma inguinale-lesion at inoculation site; hematogenous spread to bones, joints, liver

Diagnosis

biopsy of skin reveals **Donovan bodies⇒ dumbbell**-shaped en**cap**sulated rods

Chromobacterium violaceum

- inhabits soil and H_2O
- clinical-gastroenteritis after ingestion of organism; bacteremia leads to necrotic lesions in **liver**⇒all cases have resulted in **death**

Chromobacterium (chrome) violaceum (violin) del**ivers**⇒liver
results in death⇒death march

Actinobacillus actinomycetemcomitans

- normal flora mouth (sing) and intestinal tract
- causes infection in compromised (cancer) patients
- causes septicemia→leads to granulomatous lesions on several organs

Cardiobacterium hominis

- normal flora upper respiratory (nose) tract and intestine; infection in compromised patients
- bacteremia, endocarditis (♡)

Bartonella henselae

⇒ **Bar ton ella** and Hensel

- disease associated with close cat contact
- 1 week incubation; regional lymphadenopathy (>3 months); systemic symptoms rare

Diagnosis

- close cat contact; absence of bacteria in culture

Treatment

- **no antibiotics**
- **cat scratch fever**

Capnocytophaga

⇒ cap on tooth

- *C. ochracea, C. sputigena, C. gingivales*
- causes periodontal disease, bacteremia in compromised patients

Eikenella corrodens

⇒ Eek!

- normal flora of mouth and upper respiratory tract
- infections involving head and neck
- infections following human **bites**
  ⇒ better to bite

Plesiomonas shigelloides

⇒ pleasant

- natural habitat is warm surface waters and mud
- cause gastroenteritis and septicemia

Flavobacterium meningosepticum

⇒ flavored

- contaminant of **hospital** environments

Clinical

- baby→**neonatal** meningitis, bacteremia endocarditis

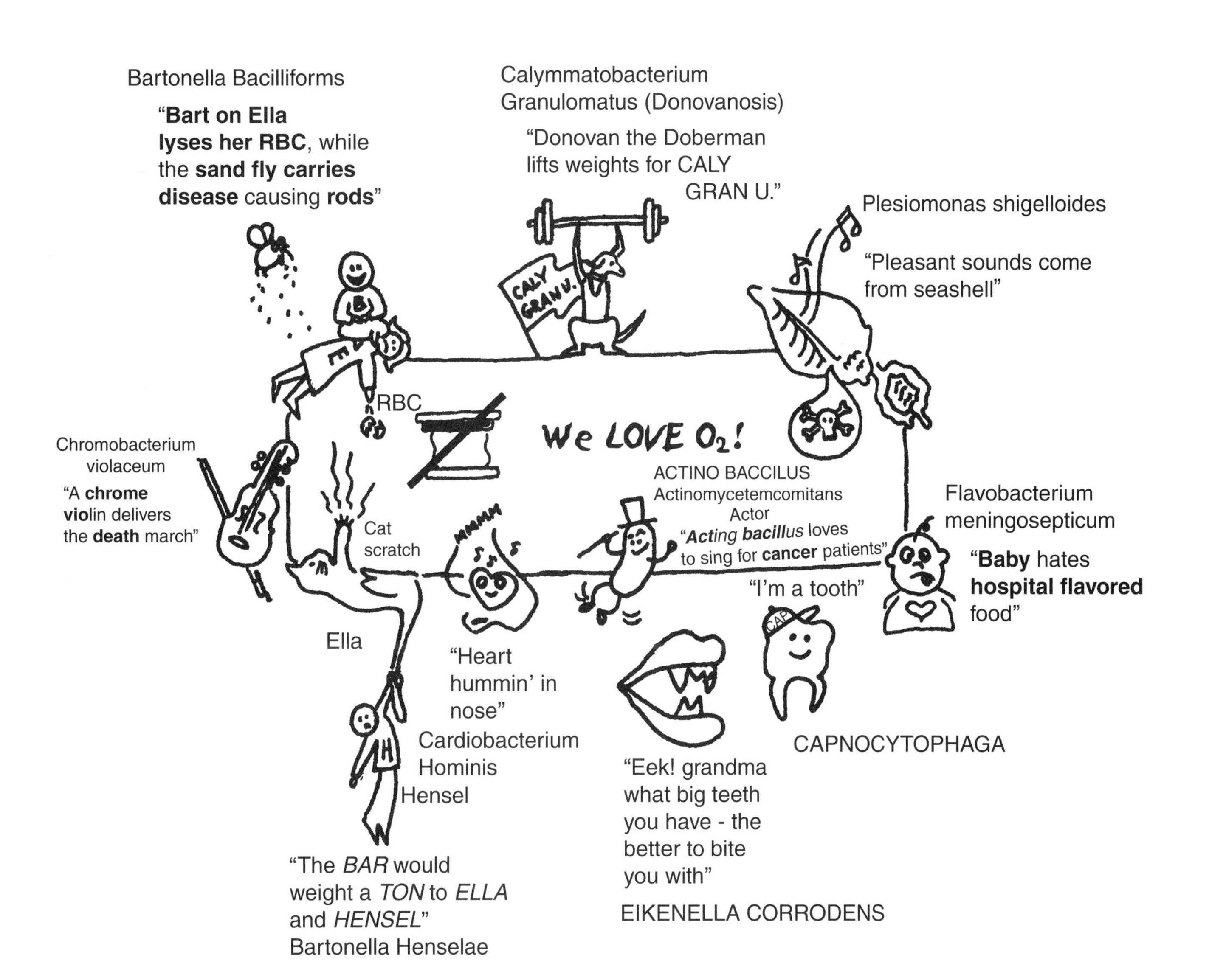
Bartonella Bacilliforms
"Bart on Ella lyses her RBC, while the sand fly carries disease causing rods"
Calymmatobacterium Granulomatus (Donovanosis)
"Donovan the Doberman lifts weights for CALY GRAN U."
CALY GRAN U.
Plesiomonas shigelloides
"Pleasant sounds come from seashell"
RBC
We LOVE O2!
Chromobacterium violaceum
"A chrome violin delivers the death march"
ACTINO BACCILUS
Actinomycetemcomitans
Actor
"Acting bacillus loves to sing for cancer patients"
Flavobacterium meningosepticum
"Baby hates hospital flavored food"
Cat scratch
"I'm a tooth"
CAP
Ella
"Heart hummin' in nose"
Cardiobacterium Hominis
Hensel
CAPNOCYTOPHAGA
"Eek! grandma what big teeth you have - the better to bite you with"
EIKENELLA CORRODENS
"The BAR would weight a TON to ELLA and HENSEL"
Bartonella Henselae

NOTES

FREQUENTLY ENCOUNTERED IN INFECTIONS

Porphyromonas

- brown-black pigmented colonies

Fusobacterium

- *Fusobacterium* **nuclea**tum: predominant species isolated from clinical material; cigar-shaped

Clostridium septicum

- isolated from patients with **malignancy**
  - ⇒ (sick in September)

Clostridium Perfringens

- most frequently isolated species
- double zone of hemolysis on blood agar

Clostridium ramosum

- 2nd most frequently isolated
- commonly resistant to antibiotics
  - ⇒ 2nd to *B. fragilis*

Prevotella

- *P. bivia*—vaginal flora; female genital tract infections

Propionibacterium

- *P. acnes*; common inhabitant of normal skin; contaminant of blood cultures

Mobiluncus

- associated with non-specific vaginitis

Actinomyces

- filamentous, pleomorphic; agent in actinomycosis
- *A. israelii, A. naeslundii*

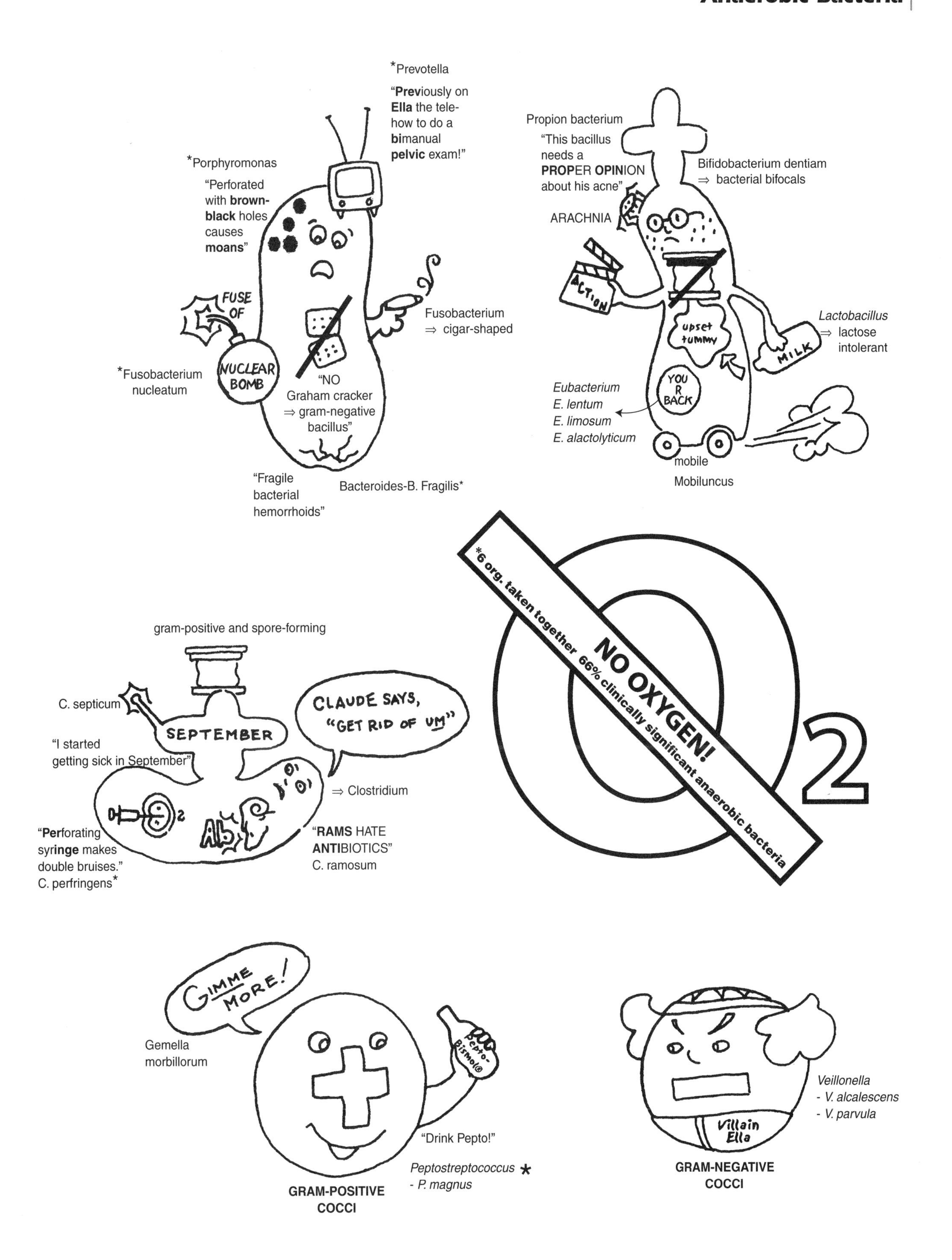
*Prevotella
"Previously on Ella the tele-how to do a bimanual pelvic exam!"
*Porphyromonas
"Perforated with brown-black holes causes moans"
FUSE OF
NUCLEAR BOMB
*Fusobacterium nucleatum
Fusobacterium
⇒ cigar-shaped
"NO Graham cracker ⇒ gram-negative bacillus"
"Fragile bacterial hemorrhoids"
Bacteroides-B. Fragilis*
Propion bacterium
"This bacillus needs a PROPER OPINION about his acne"
Bifidobacterium dentiam
⇒ bacterial bifocals
ARACHNIA
ACTION
upset tummy
MILK
Lactobacillus
⇒ lactose intolerant
YOU R BACK
Eubacterium
E. lentum
E. limosum
E. alactolyticum
mobile
Mobiluncus
NO OXYGEN!
*6 org. taken together 66% clinically significant anaerobic bacteria
O2
gram-positive and spore-forming
C. septicum
SEPTEMBER
"I started getting sick in September"
CLAUDE SAYS, "GET RID OF UM"
⇒ Clostridium
"Perforating syringe makes double bruises."
C. perfringens*
Ab
"RAMS HATE ANTIBIOTICS"
C. ramosum
GIMME MORE!
Gemella morbillorum
Pepto-Bismol®
"Drink Pepto!"
Peptostreptococcus *
- P. magnus
GRAM-POSITIVE COCCI
Villain Ella
Veillonella
- V. alcalescens
- V. parvula
GRAM-NEGATIVE COCCI

⇒ Claude says, "get rid of um!"

CLOSTRIDIUM

C. difficile-cause of antibiotic-associated intestinal disease

- antimicrobials that can induce disease: ampicillin, clindamycin, cephalosporins; disruption of intestinal flora by antimicrobial agent→*C. difficile* colonizes tract→multiplies and releases 2 toxins→enterotoxin A and cytotoxin B; causes wide spectrum of intestinal diseases→complications: toxic megacolon, perforation of bowel; death

Diagnosis

Sigmoidoscopy→demonstration of pseudomembrane

- demonstration of toxin in stool specimen

Treatment

Discontinue antimicrobial agent; vancomycin, bacitracin, and metronidazole eliminates *C. difficile* from intestinal tract

CLOSTRIDIAL MYONECROSIS (GAS GANGRENE)

- gas gangrene characterized by extensive necrosis of muscle and overlying soft tissue
- caused by: *C. perfringens* (most cases), *C. septicum, C. novyi, C. bifermentans*
- usually mixed infection—aerobic/anaerobic and more than one species of *Clostridium*

NOTES

Pathogenesis

- traumatic myonecrosis, non-traumatic or (spontaneous) myonecrosis→bowel leakage from carcinoma, uterine gas gangrene→species multiply in wound→elaborate potent exotoxins—(α-toxin) lecithinase closely associated with virulence→rapid and progressive destruction of tissue

Diagnosis

Gram stain (with few neutrophils)→isolation and identification→*C. perfringens*—double zone of hemolysis on blood agar and lecithinase production and neutralization with antitoxin to α-toxin

Treatment

surgical debridement, antimicrobial agents (penicillin), gas gangrene antitoxin, hyperbaric O_2

C. PERFRINGENS (FOOD POISONING)

- causes 2 different food poisonings
  - ⇒ enterocolitis and *Enteritis necroticans*

Enterocolitis

- *C. perfringens type A* is etiologic agent also *Staphylococcusaureus* and *Salmonella*
- meats and gravies usually involved

Pathogenesis

ingestion→multiplication→ sporulation in intestinal tract→release of enterotoxin (heat labile protein which is part of the spore coat)→watery diarrhea and abdominal pain

Diagnosis

symptoms and isolation in patients' stools

Treatment

none because short duration and not life-threatening

Enteritis Necroticans

- *C. perfringens* type C is the etiologic agent: principally in *highlands of New Guinea*

Pathogenesis

from undercooked pork→β-toxin is released in small intestine causing necrosis with high mortality

- predisposing factors—↓ intestinal proteolytic activity; staple diet of sweet potatoes (trypsin inhibitor)
- no treatment because such rapid course; vaccine (β-toxin) effective

C. BOTULINUM

- paralytic disease; not infectious disease but intoxication
- ⇒ toxin produced outside the body and is ingested
- *C. botulinum* does not invade tissue
- spores can withstand boiling for several hours
- predominant exposure comes from food; improperly home canned or home prepared foods; undercooked fish
- botulinum toxin (neurotoxin)—prevents neurotransmission by preventing release *of* Acetylcholine; 8 toxins produced (A, B, C_1, C_2, D, E, F, G); all same mechanism of action; presence of bacteriophage required for toxin production; heat labile; most potent toxin known to humans

Pathogenesis

- food poisoning—ingest toxin→toxin to nerve endings through bloodstream→ cranial nerves affected first→then descending paralysis
- wound botulism; infant botulism→spores ingested (honey)→toxin produced in intestinal tract→infant first constipated then becomes weaker→"floppy baby syndrome"→one cause of SIDS→no natural immunity

Diagnosis

demonstration of toxin

Treatment

antitoxin→only neutralizes circulating toxin; penicillin; therapeutic uses of neurotoxin: dystonias and strabismus

C. TETANI (TETANUS)

- gram-positive with terminal swollen spores
- resembles tennis racket or drumstick

Pathogenesis

wound contamination (spores)→other organism ↓ O_2; multiplies locally produces tetanospasmin (neurotoxin)→blocks release of inhibitory neuro transmitter→nerves fired continuously resulting in spasmodic contractions

- clinical: generalized tetanus (most)→"Risus sardonicus"—1st symptom→contraction of facial muscles→contractions then spread through host
- localized tetanus—cephalic tetanus→results from injury to the head→may progress into generalized tetanus
- tetanus neonatorum→infection of umbilicus
- death—due to asphyxiation as a result of contraction of respiratory muscles or cardiac failure
- active/natural immunity

Diagnosis

Gram stain

Treatment

debridements of wound antitoxin→inactivates unbound toxin; antimicrobials (*penicillin*)

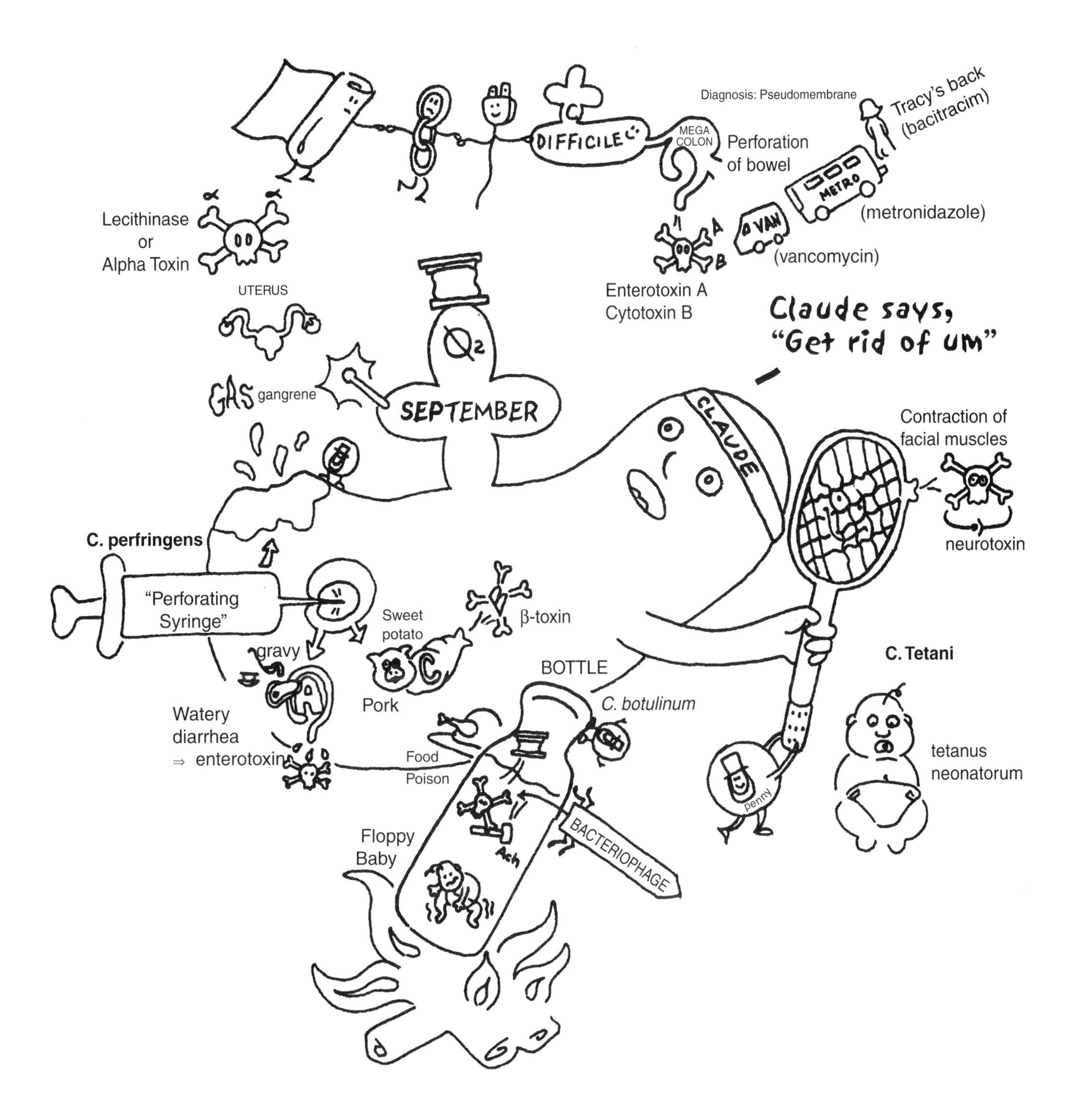
Diagnosis: Pseudomembrane
Tracy's back
(bacitracim)
DIFFICILE
MEGA COLON
Perforation
of bowel
METRO
(metronidazole)
VAN
(vancomycin)
A
B
Enterotoxin A
Cytotoxin B
Lecithinase
or
Alpha Toxin
UTERUS
O2
GAS gangrene
SEPTEMBER
Claude says,
"Get rid of um"
CLAUDE
Contraction of
facial muscles
neurotoxin
C. perfringens
"Perforating
Syringe"
Sweet
potato
β-toxin
gravy
Pork
BOTTLE
C. botulinum
C. Tetani
Watery
diarrhea
⇒ enterotoxin
Food
Poison
Ach
penny
tetanus
neonatorum
Floppy
Baby
BACTERIOPHAGE

ACTINOMYCETES

⇒ "Action, Mice Eat"

ACTINOMYCOSIS

- caused by *Actinomyces israelii*
  - ⇒ star of David
- anaerobe which is part of normal flora of oral cavity
- local trauma allows infection to occur and sulfur granules (hard yellow granules⇒ star of David points colored yellow) form in pus
- drains pus through sinus tracts
- abscess formation in cervicofacial (most common), thoracic, and abdominal areas; non-communicable
- diagnosis: 1) identification of gram (+) rods (branching) with sulfur granules
- treatment with penicillin G⇒penny with G sign; surgical drainage

NOCARDIOSIS

⇒ no cardio (no heart)

- caused by *Nocardia asteroides*
  - ⇒ "asteriod with no heart about to crash mice"
- aerobes found in soil (gram-positive)
- immunocompromised in danger of dissemination after initial lung infection
- weakly acid-fast
- non-communicable

Diagnosis

identification of gram (+) rods that are weakly acid-fast

Treatment

trimethoprim-sulfamethoxazole (co-trimoxazole)

⇒ dog on cot's rim→refer to folic acid inhibitors drawing for explanation

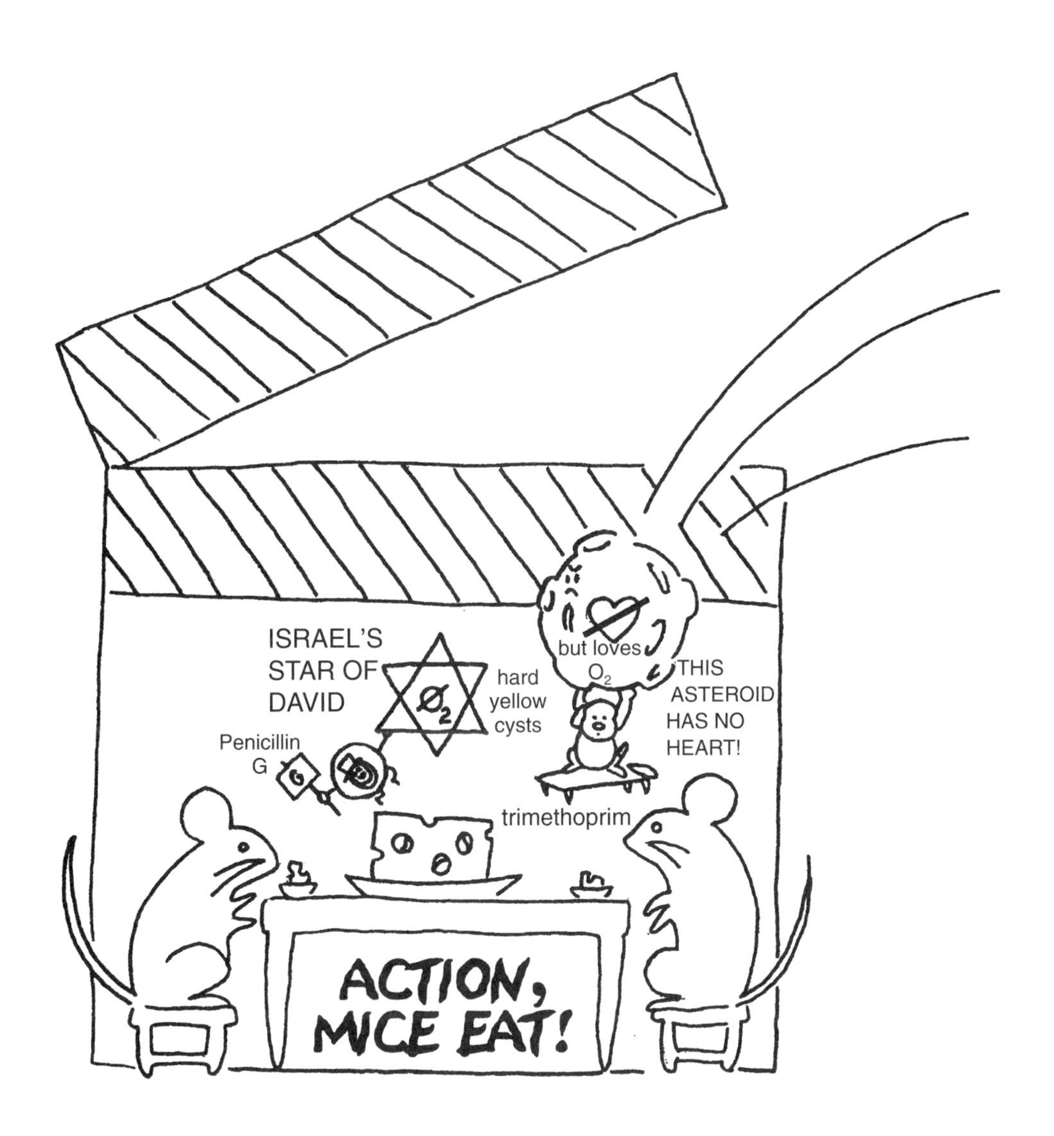
ISRAEL'S
STAR OF
DAVID
$\not{O}_2$
hard
yellow
cysts
but loves
O_2
THIS
ASTEROID
HAS NO
HEART!
Penicillin
G
trimethoprim
ACTION,
MICE EAT!

III. MYCOLOGY

NOTES

GENERAL ANTIFUNGALS

⇒ Anti Fun Gal

IMIDAZOLES AND TRIAZOLES

- inhibit C P450 and ergosterol biosynthesis

Imidazoles

ketoconazole⇒key on toe
- topical and oral

clotrimazole⇒clown trims
- topical

miconazole⇒microphone
- topical and IV

Triazoles

itraconazole⇒"I train lions"
- used on nails to treat **f**ungus
- oral

fluconazole⇒flute
- *oral* and *IV*

econazole⇒E on engine
- inhibition of ergosterol biosynthesis
- topical treatment for dermatophytosis, pityriasis versicolor, cutaneous candidiasis

butaconazole⇒butt with O
- treats vaginal candidiasis
- topical

terconazole⇒turkey
- treats vaginal candidiasis
- topical

oxiconazole⇒Ox
- treats dermatophytosis
- topical

sulconazole⇒sulking
- treats dermatophytosis
- topical

tioconazole⇒tie with O
- treats vaginal candidiasis
- topical

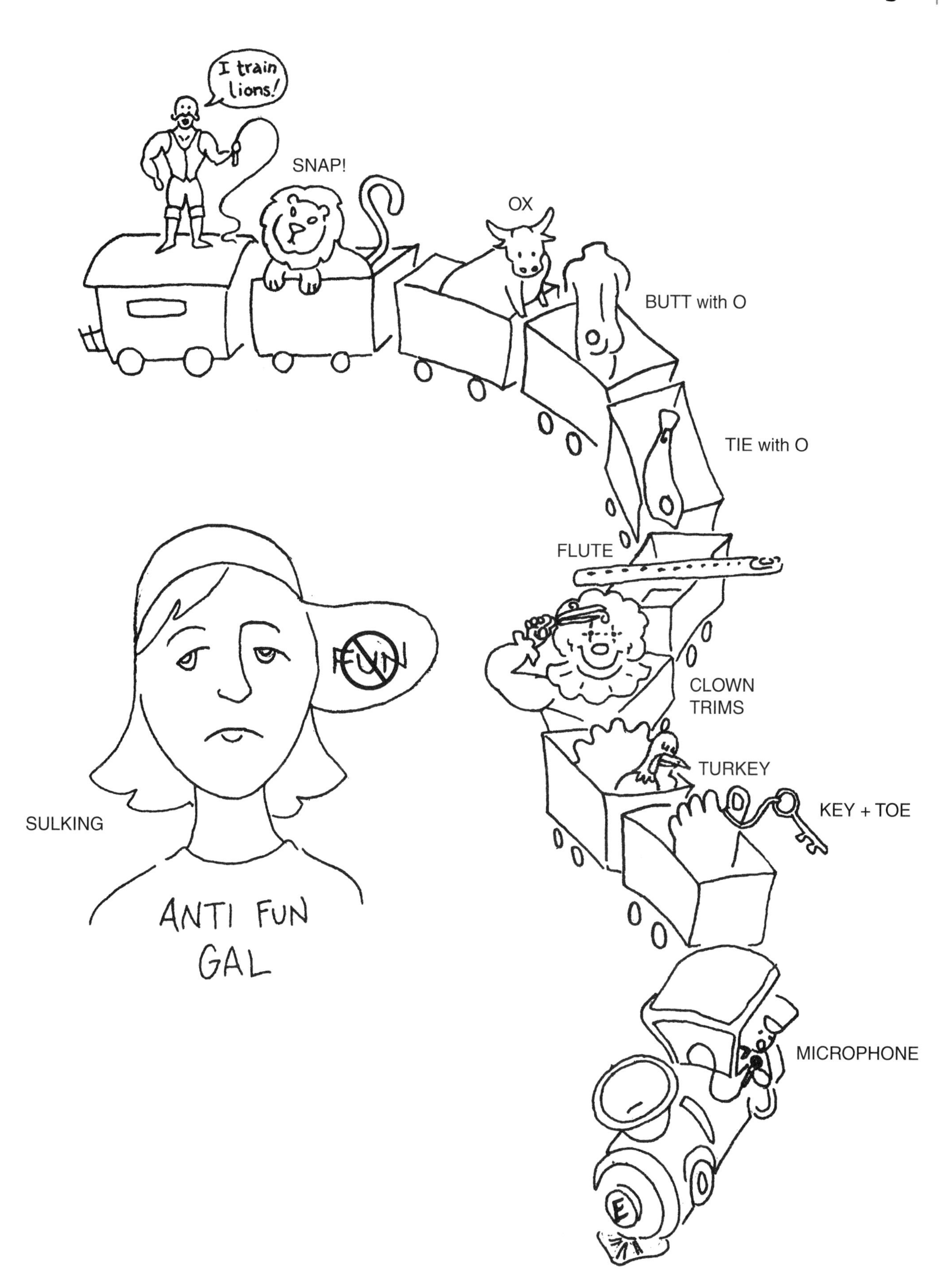
I train lions!
SNAP!
OX
BUTT with O
TIE with O
FLUTE
CLOWN TRIMS
TURKEY
KEY + TOE
MICROPHONE
SULKING
FUN
ANTI FUN GAL
E

NOTES

TOPICAL ANTIFUNGALS

⇒ tropical tree

Haloprogin⇒halo and grin
- treats dermatophytosis and cutaneous candidiasis
- prescription

Undecylenic acid and zinc undecylenate⇒ undies and *acid*

- used to treat dermatophytosis such as athlete's foot
- MOA: affects fungal membrane formation and function; OTC

Ciclopirox Olamine

⇒ cyclone and pie of rocks (rox)
- treats dermatophytosis and cutaneous candidiasis
- interferes with uptake of K^+ and amino acids by fungus
- prescription

Squalene 2,3-epoxidase inhibitors⇒"*squaw leaning*"

Tolnaftate⇒toll booth
- used to treat dermatophytosis; OTC

Naftifine⇒NAFTA agreement
- used to treat dermatophytosis; prescription

Terbinafine⇒turban
- an allylamine
- used to treat dermatophytosis; prescription

Butenafine⇒**Boo ten** times!
- used to treat dermatophytosis; prescription

Clioquinol⇒*Cleopatra*
- treats dermatophytosis

Triacetin

⇒ 3 aces in tin
- treats dermatophytosis
- OTC

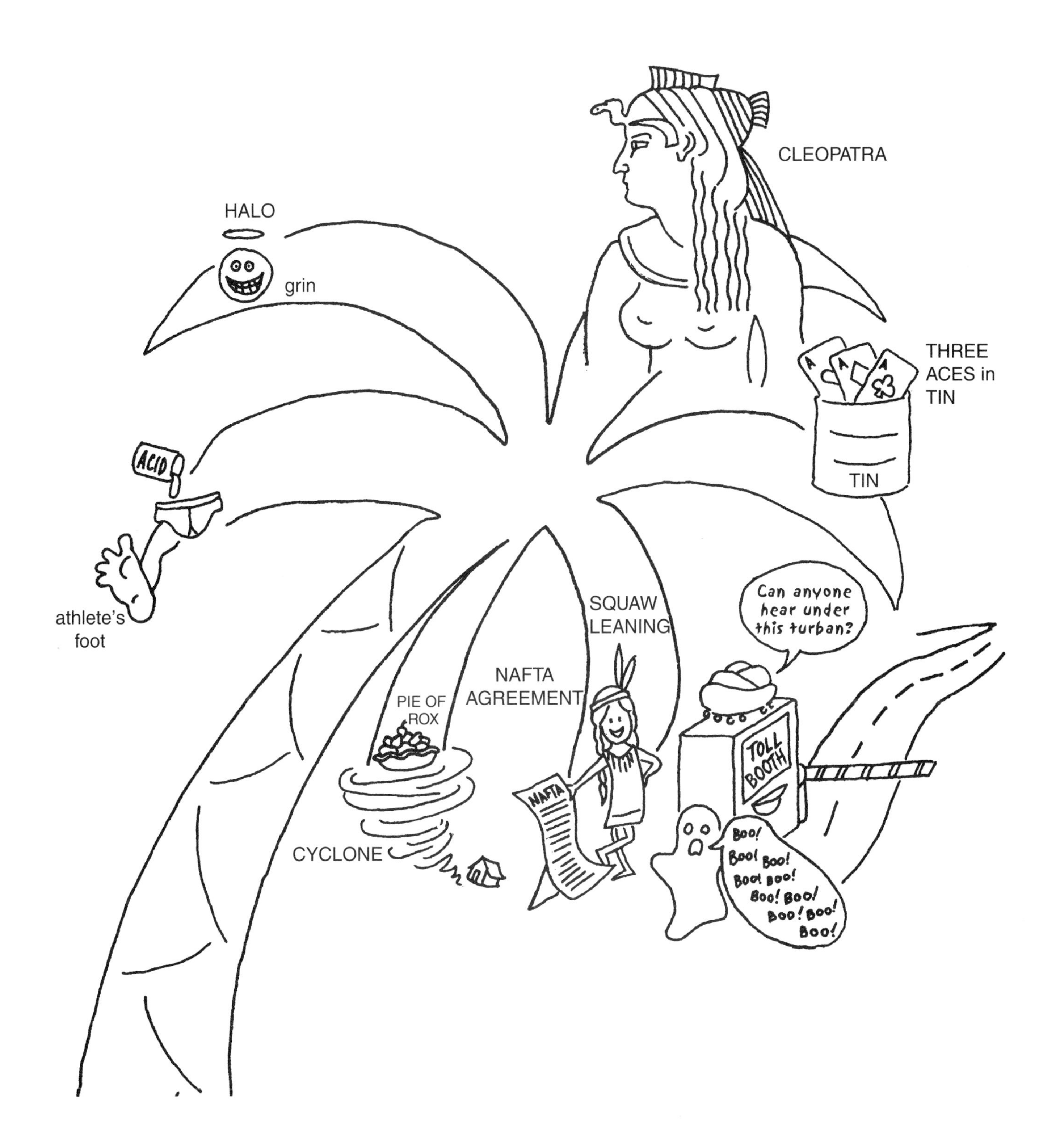
CLEOPATRA
HALO
grin
THREE ACES in TIN
TIN
ACID
athlete's foot
SQUAW LEANING
Can anyone hear under this turban?
NAFTA AGREEMENT
PIE OF ROX
TOLL BOOTH
NAFTA
CYCLONE
Boo! Boo! Boo! Boo! Boo! Boo! Boo! Boo! Boo! Boo!

NOTES

ORAL ANTIFUNGALS

griseofulvin⇒grizzly bear
- used for dermatophytosis
- binds to keratin and disrupts mitotic spindle interfering with normal mitosis

5-fluorocytosine⇒flower with 5 petals
- used for cryptococcal candida infections
- interferes with protein synthesis
- fungal resistance can develop

echinocandin/pneumocandin⇒echinoderm with candy
- systemic and opportunistic infections
- B(1, 3) glucan biosynthesis inhibitors

Nikkomycin *Z*⇒Nike symbol
- treat systemic and opportunistic infections
- inhibits chitin biosynthesis

POLYENES

nystatin⇒N.Y. Staten Island
- topical fungicidal used to treat cutaneous candidiasis
- alters membrane function by binding ergosterol

amphotericin B⇒amp with B on it
- used to treat systemic and opportunistic infections
- alters membrane function by binding ergosterol
- nephrotoxic
- liposomal amphotericin B complexed with lipids to increase speed of drug action and also reduces toxicity

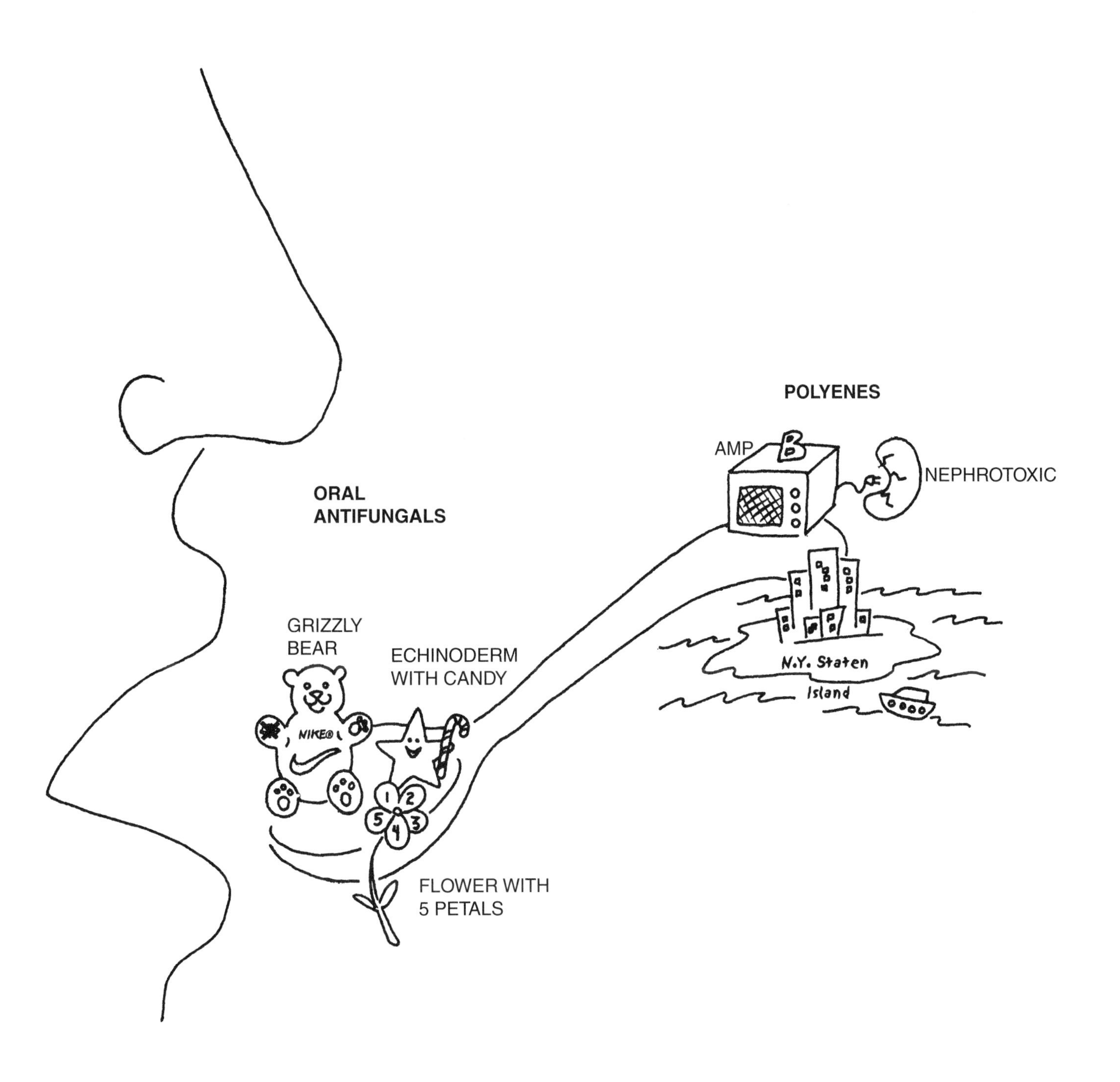
POLYENES
AMP
B
NEPHROTOXIC
ORAL
ANTIFUNGALS
N.Y. Staten
Island
GRIZZLY
BEAR
NIKE®
ECHINODERM
WITH CANDY
1
2
3
4
5
FLOWER WITH
5 PETALS

NOTES

CUTANEOUS MYCOSES

Tinea Nigra

⇒ Tiny Niagara Falls
- infection of kerantinized layers of skin
- hyphae pigment causes **brownish spots**
- caused by *Cladosporium werneckii* which is found in soil and transmitted during injury
- found in southern states
- treated with **topical** (tropical tree) **keratolytic** (carrots) agent

Tinea versicolor (pityriasis versicolor)

⇒ pitiful sis
⇒ versatile colors
- superficial skin infection
- considered a problem for cosmetic reasons only
- caused by **Malassezia furfur**
  ⇒ pouring molasses on furry chest
- hypopigmented lesions which occur more often in hot humid weather
- lesions contain budding⇒(buddin' bread) yeast cells and hypha⇒(hyphen) which can be observed when skin scrapings, from lesions, are mixed with KOH
- treat with miconazole⇒(microphone)

SUBCUTANEOUS MYCOSES

SOIL and vegetation fungus are first introduced into subcutaneous layer through trauma

Chromomycosis

⇒ chromosomes
- several fungi cause
- appears as slowly progressive granulomatous infection
- dematiaceous because of melanin-like pigment production
- found in tropics
- lesions appear along lymphatics
- brown fungal cells are found in leukocytes or giant cells
- treat with oral flucytosine or thiabendazole

Mycetoma

⇒ mice toe
- pus from lesions contains compact colored granules
- similar lesions to actinomycetes
- no effective drug treatment

Sporotrichosis

⇒ **spo**iled **rot**ten, **rich**
- dimorphic fungus that lives on vegetation
- *Sporothrix schenckii* is dimorphic
  ⇒ tissue specimen will have **cigar**-shaped budding yeasts
  ⇒ in culture there will be hyphae with conidia clusters resembling **daisies**
- may cause local pustule or draining lymphatics may contain ulcers with nodules
- treat with itraconazole or oral potassium iodide

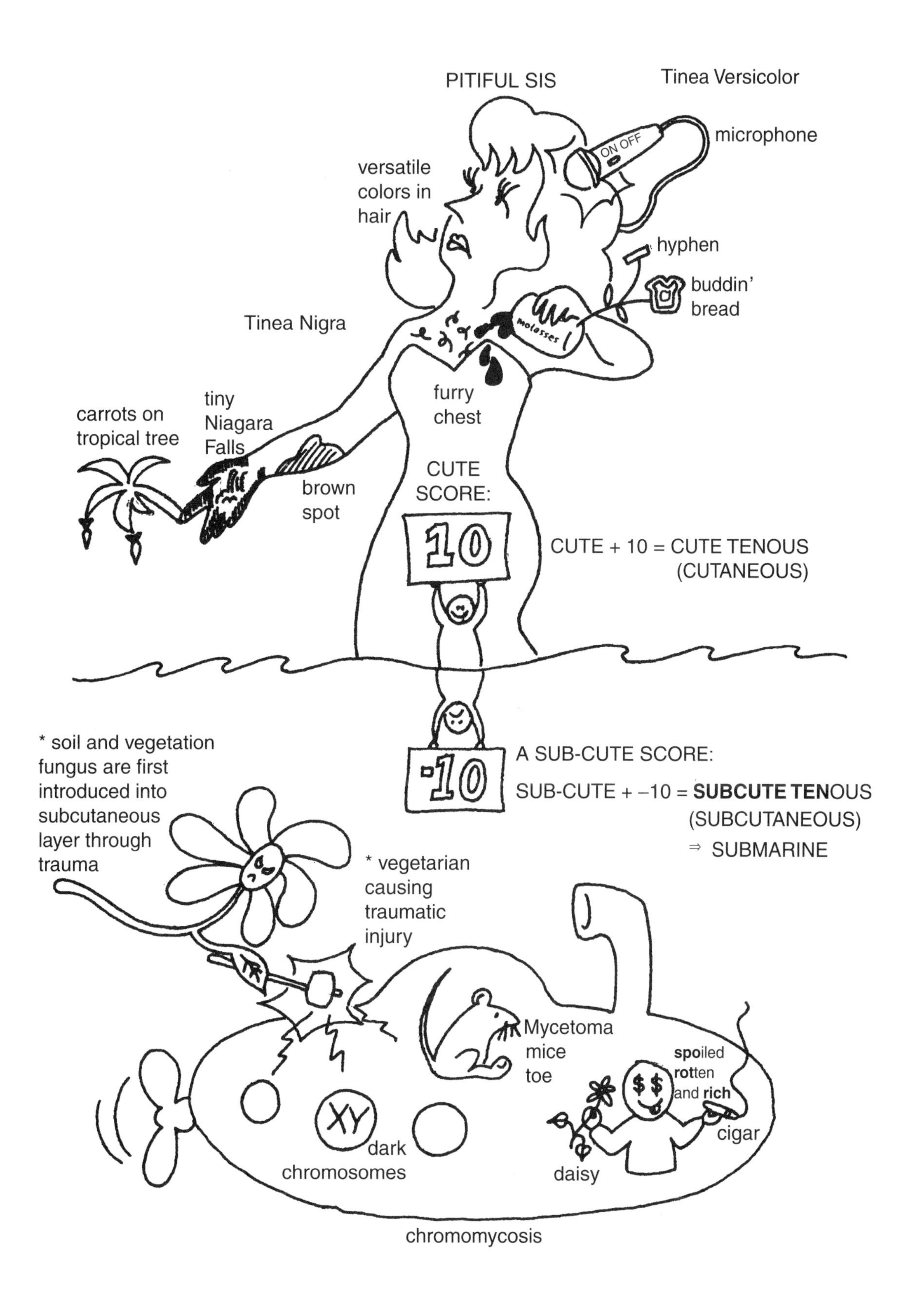
PITIFUL SIS
Tinea Versicolor
ON OFF
microphone
versatile colors in hair
hyphen
buddin' bread
Tinea Nigra
molasses
furry chest
carrots on tropical tree
tiny Niagara Falls
brown spot
CUTE SCORE:
10
CUTE + 10 = CUTE TENOUS (CUTANEOUS)
-10
A SUB-CUTE SCORE:
SUB-CUTE + –10 = SUBCUTE TENOUS (SUBCUTANEOUS)
⇒ SUBMARINE
* soil and vegetation fungus are first introduced into subcutaneous layer through trauma
* vegetarian causing traumatic injury
Mycetoma mice toe
spoiled rotten and rich
XY
dark chromosomes
daisy
cigar
chromomycosis

NOTES

GENERAL CHARACTERISTICS

- infection results from inhalation (lungs) of spores (smores)
- dimorphic: found as mold in soil and yeast in tissue (or spherule) such as lungs
- no person-to-person transmission

PARACOCCIDIOIDES

⇒ pair of cocci

- caused by *P. brasiliensis* (South American blastomycosis)
- dimorphic: mold in soil and yeast in tissue
- yeast is thick-walled with many buds as shown →
- endemic in Latin America
- microscopically, from pus or tissue samples, yeast cells with multiple buds can be seen
- treat with itraconazole

COCCIDIOIDES

⇒ caused by *C. immitis*
⇒ coccus

- dimorphic fungus
  - ⇒ mold in soil and spherule (sphere) in tissue
- endemic in southwest United States and Latin America
  - ⇒ Lower **Sonoran Life Zone** (snoring)
- in soil the fungus forms hyphae with alternating arthrospores
- dissemination occurs once spores have infected the lungs
  - ⇒ organs affected are primarily bones and CNS where granulomatous lesions form
- dissemination occurs in individuals with compromised cell-mediated immunity
- clinical findings include fever and cough; lung damage; erythema nodosum or arthralgias (a.k.a. valley fever in California) and (a.k.a. desert rheumatism in Arizona)
- no organisms in lesions

Diagnosis

tissue specimen with spherules; positive skin test

Treatment

1. amphotericin B—chronic lung lesions or disseminated disease
2. ketoconazole—lung disease
3. fluconazole—meningitis

HISTOPLASMA

⇒ His (♂) toe

- caused by *H. capsulatum*
- mold in soil; yeast in tissue
- two types of asexual spores
  1) tuberculate macroconidia
  2) microconidia→infective when inhaled
- endemic in central and eastern United States (Ohio and Mississippi River Valleys)
- transmitted by bat guano and where soil is heavily contaminated with bird droppings (birds are not infected, however)
- clinical findings include oval budding yeast inside macrophages; pneumonia may develop with extensive exposure; AIDS patients and those with reduced CMI are particularly at risk; AIDS patients will develop ulcerated lesions on tongue

Diagnosis

⇒ tissue—oval budding yeast cell in macrophage
⇒ culture—hyphae with tuberculate macroconidia

Treatment

1. oral itraconazole—progressive lung lesions
2. amphotericin B—disseminated disease

BLASTOMYCES

- caused by *B. dermatitidis* (North American blastomycosis)
- dimorphic: mold in soil; yeast in tissue
- yeast cell is broad-based bud
- endemic in eastern United States, but occurs in other parts of the world also
- in soil, you will find hyphae with pear-shaped conidia
- conidia infective once inhaled
- dissemination results in ulcerated granulomas (skin, bone, etc.)
- treat with itraconazole or amphotericin B

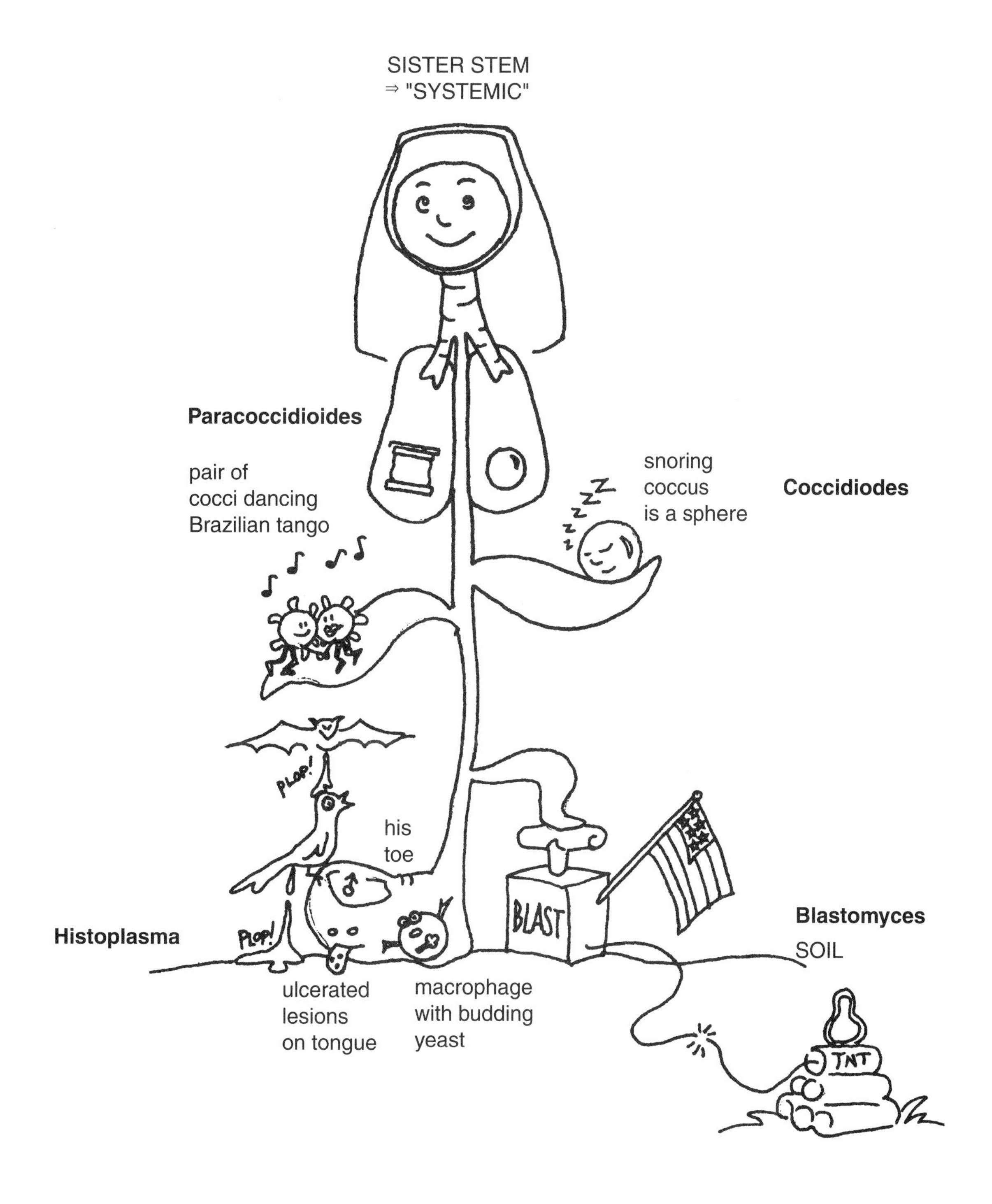
SISTER STEM
⇒ "SYSTEMIC"
Paracoccidioides
pair of
cocci dancing
Brazilian tango
snoring
coccus
is a sphere
Coccidiodes
PLOP!
his
toe
BLAST
Histoplasma
PLOP!
ulcerated
lesions
on tongue
macrophage
with budding
yeast
Blastomyces
SOIL
TNT

Opportunistic Mycoses (Opera Tune)

NOTES

ASPERGILLUS

⇒ asp

- *A. fumigatus* (fumes rising from asp) cause infections of skin, eye, ears; "fungus ball" in lungs and allergic bronchopulmonary aspergillosis
- exist only as molds
- septate hyphae with V-shaped branches
- form radiating chains
- transmission from airborne *Candida*
- most common cause of fungal sinusitis
- diagnosis made from specimens with septate branching hyphae

Treatment

invasive Aspergillus—amphotericin B

CRYPTOCOCCUS

⇒ crypt of coccus

- *C. neoformans* (foreman) causes cryptococcus
- most common life-threatening fungal infection in AIDS patients
- oval, budding yeast in wide polysaccharide capsule⇒cap with wide brim
- grows in soil where bird (pigeon) droppings are
- infection from inhalation

Diagnosis

- use India ink to identify in CSF; CSF→high titer of capsular antigen→detected by latex particle agglutination test

Treatment

1) meningitis and disseminated disease→combined therapy of amphotericin B and flucytosine
2) long-term suppression of meningitis in AIDS patients—fluconazole

MUCOR AND RHIZOPUS

⇒ core says moo ⇒ rising pus

- cause mucormycosis
- saprophytic molds
- not dimorphic
- transmitted by airborne asexual spores
- grow in blood vessel walls and cause infarction and necrosis of distal tissue
- diabetics with ketoacidosis particularly susceptible

Diagnosis

- specimens with nonseptate hyphae; broad, irregular walls; branches form at right angles

Treatment

- amphotericin B and surgery

CANDIDA

⇒ Canada

- *Candida albicans* causes thrush, vaginitis, and chronic mucocutaneous candidiasis
- oval yeast with single bud
- part of normal flora of GI, upper respiratory tract, and female genital tracts
- in tissue appears as pseudohyphae
- not transmitted since part of normal flora already
- disease results when immune system compromised

Diagnosis

1) pseudohyphae and budding yeast seen
2) *C. albicans* form germ tubes at 37° in serum
3) *C. albican* forms chlamydospores

Treatment

1) thrush—fluconazole
2) skin infections—topical antifungals
3) mucocutaneous candidiasis—ketoconazole
4) disseminated candidiasis—amphotericin B or fluconazole

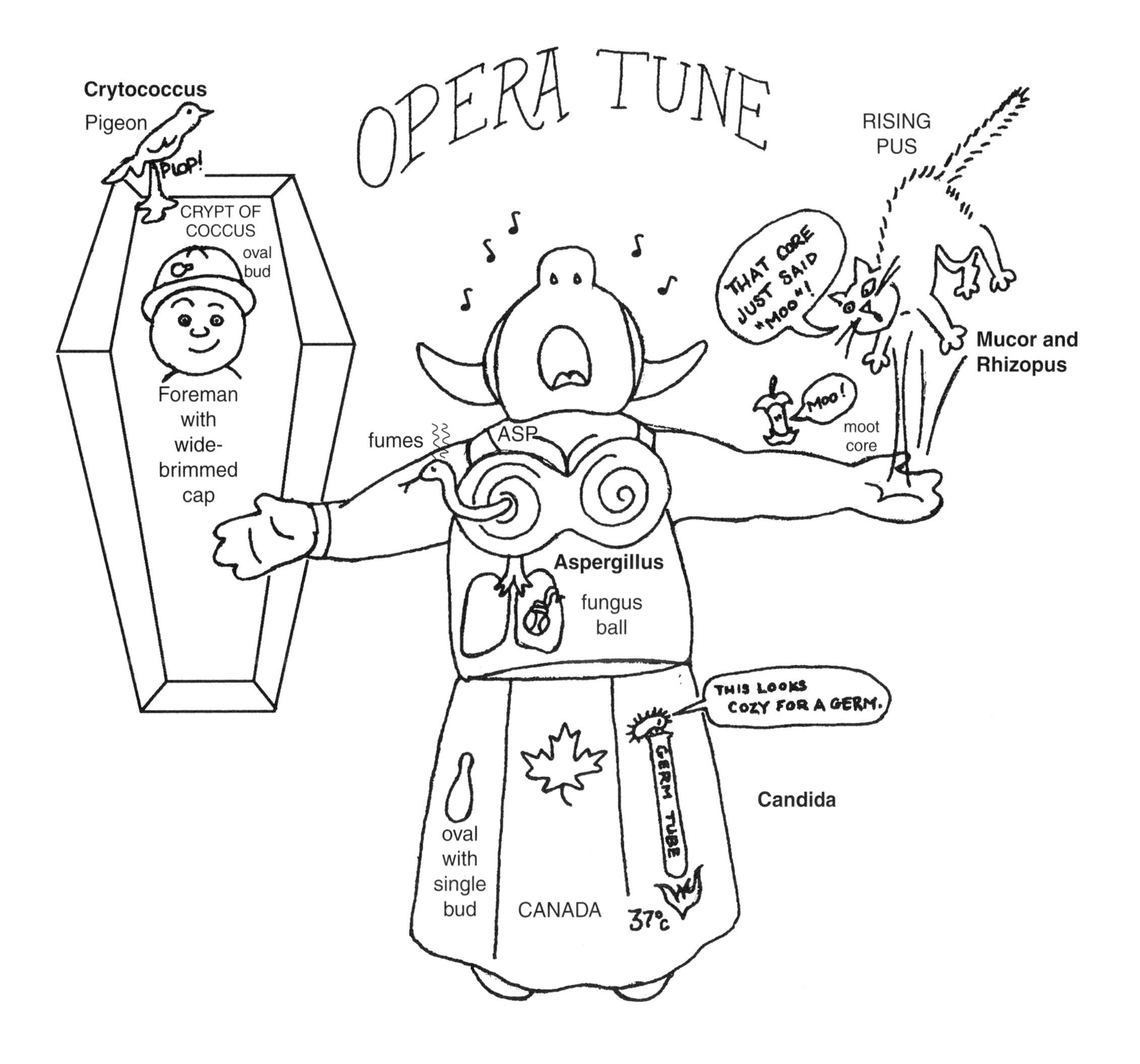
OPERA TUNE
Crytococcus
Pigeon
PLOP!
CRYPT OF COCCUS
oval bud
Foreman with wide-brimmed cap
RISING PUS
THAT CORE JUST SAID "MOO"!
Mucor and Rhizopus
MOO!
moot core
fumes
ASP
Aspergillus
fungus ball
THIS LOOKS COZY FOR A GERM.
GERM TUBE
Candida
oval with single bud
CANADA
37°c

IV.
VIROLOGY

NOTES

immunotherapy

- immunoglobulins:
  - ⇒ (passive vaccine): hepatitis B and A, chickenpox, rabies, measles; interferon-α-2b: HPV, HCV

Protease Inhibitors

- pharmacophores compete with viral polypeptides for the protease and bind irreversibly to it
- **indi**navir, **rit**onavir, **saq**uinavir
- MOA: prevent post-translational cleavage of GAG and GAG-Pol polypeptides that is essential for maturation of the virion: without cleavage immature non-infectious particles bud from membrane
- spectrum: HIV

Viral Reverse Transcriptase (⊥/H) Nonnucleoside Inhibitors

⇒ "no nuclear war"

nevirapine—"nevi→mole"

⇒ MOA: binds away from **active** site of RT (**nevi is away from activist's active mouth**)

but prevents catalyst needed to incorporate base into growing chain; alters cleavage specificity of RNase H activity of RT;

- spectrum: **HIV**

Ion Channel Blockers

- amantadine→"Amen to dine"
- MOA: inhibits **M-Z** capsid protein from functioning→↑ pH (basically) of viral endosome→blocks conformational change in hemaglutinin (HA) required for fusion of membranes; prevents HA from assuming correct conformation for incorporation into budding virion
- spectrum: influenza A (fly with A wings), Parkinson's disease (causes dopamine release from intact nerve terminals)
- toxicity: slurred speech, ataxia, dizziness

Viral Reverse Transcriptase (RT) or RNA-Dependent DNA Polymerase Nucleoside Analogues

⇒ nuclear explosion

- **zid**ovudine⇒(AZT) (zipper): enters as prodrug→host cell phosphorylates AZT to AZT-TP→incorporated into growing DNA chain in place of thymidine-TP→ terminating it
- AZT-TP also ↓ cellular thymidine kinase so adenosine-TP levels ↓; **AZT only inhibits replication not infection**
- spectrum: HIV⇒"HIVE"

Viral DNA-Dependent DNAP Nucleoside Analogues

modified bases trick the viral DNAP into binding the analogue, which results in premature chain termination

- acyclovir (ACV) enters cell as prodrug→herpes virus thymidine kinase phosphorylates ACV→ACV-monophosphate (ACV-MP)→cellular guanosine-MP kinase→ACV-MP to ACV-TP (active)→ ACV-TP into chain→termination chain elongation "**v**iral **h**and**s**hake"→**HS**V-1, **HS**V-2, ⇒VZV, EBV ganciclovir→CMV
- (cretinitis in HIV patients)
- fluorouracil→HPV (genital warts)
  - ⇒ "flower with human face"

Viral DNAP, RT Inhibitors Pyrophosphate Analogues

⇒ "pirate hat on fox"

- bind to pyrophosphate-binding site of DNAP or RT and block dNTP binding
- foscarnet→spectrum: HIV (**hive**);

HBV (**h**am**b**urger); CMV (**see me** gi**v**e); HSV 1 and 2 (**h**and**s**hake)

toxicity: can inhibit cellular DNA replication in kidney and bone marrow

Inhibition of Viral RNA or DNA Replication by Blocking Important Vital Enzymes→"Virus End"

ribavirin→"ribbon"

- ⇒ must be phosphorylated (1, 2, or 3)
- ⇒ ribavirin-MP→inhibits cellular **inosine** 5′ (I know sign)-5′-MP-OH→depleting GTP
- ⇒ ribavirin-TP→interferes with 5′ capping of mRNAs by inhibiting cellular guanylyl transferase
- ⇒ ribavirin-MP, DP, or TP→directly inhibit viral RNA-dependent RNAP

spectrum for IV—Lassa fever virus, Hantaan virus; aerosol—RSV

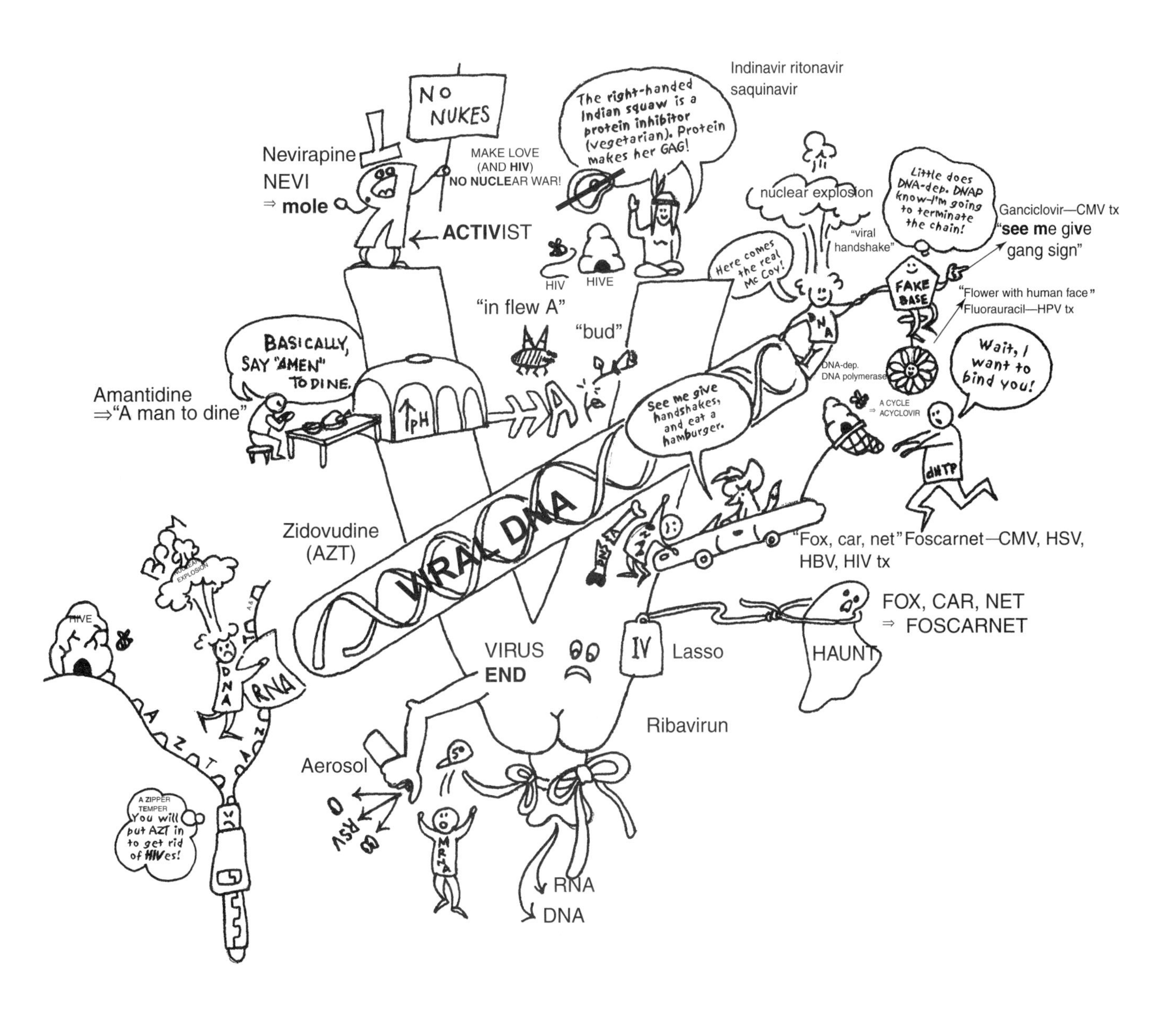
Indinavir ritonavir saquinavir
NO NUKES
The right-handed Indian squaw is a protein inhibitor (vegetarian). Protein makes her GAG!
Nevirapine
NEVI
⇒ mole
MAKE LOVE (AND HIV) NO NUCLEAR WAR!
ACTIVIST
nuclear explosion
"viral handshake"
Little does DNA-dep. DNAP know–I'm going to terminate the chain!
Ganciclovir—CMV tx
"see me give gang sign"
HIV
HIVE
Here comes the real Mc Coy!
FAKE BASE
"Flower with human face"
Fluorauracil—HPV tx
"in flew A"
"bud"
BASICALLY, SAY "AMEN" TO DINE.
Amantidine
⇒"A man to dine"
pH
DNA-dep. DNA polymerase
Wait, I want to bind you!
A CYCLE ⇒ ACYCLOVIR
See me give handshakes, and eat a hamburger.
dNTP
VIRAL DNA
Zidovudine (AZT)
"Fox, car, net" Foscarnet—CMV, HSV, HBV, HIV tx
FOX, CAR, NET
⇒ FOSCARNET
HIVE
RNA
DNA
VIRUS
END
IV
Lasso
HAUNT
Ribavirun
Aerosol
RSV
A ZIPPER TEMPER
You will put AZT in to get rid of HIVes!
RNA
DNA

NOTES

ADENOVIRIDAE

⇒ "add in no votes!"

- *General*: CPE in tonsils and adenoids; dsDNA with linear genome with terminal protein attached to the 5′ end of each strand→this protein, together with a CMP molecule, serves as the primer for DNA replication
- icosahedral and non-enveloped; each penton contains fiber that serves as the viral attachment protein and acts as a hemagglutinin (HA)
- infect the respiratory tract, eye, bladder, and intestines

Replicative Cycle

Viral fiber reacts with cell surface receptors and virus enters the host cell by endocytosis→
capsid delivers genome to nucleus→
replication

⇒ early proteins replicate first (also small RNA)→genome→late proteins effect on host cell→no DNA and RNA replicate; **paracrystalline arrays (inclusion bodies)** found in host cell nucleus

Pathogenesis

acquisition primary fecal/oral; replicates at point of entry

- in immunocompromised→disseminate by viremia affecting the skin and visceral organs
- productive infection→focal necrosis due to toxic penton fibers→(shut down macromolecule synthesis) and immune-mediated damage to infected cell
- latent infection persists years in lymphoid tissue

Proteins Encoded by Genome

E1A—activates viral gene transcription, binds cellular growth suppressor RB; deregulates cell growth; inhibits activation of INF
E1B—binds cellular growth suppressor p53; inhibits apoptosis
E2—promotor activator (DNA binding proteins); terminal protein attached to DNA; DNAP
E3—protection from immune response; inhibits TNF-α cytotoxic
E4—binds MHC-1 heavy chain preventing membrane expression
VA RNA_I, VA RNA_{II}—inhibits cellular protein kinase (antiviral state)

Epidemiology

stable in environment, resistant to drying, detergents, acids, proteases, bile, mild chlorination

- easily spread by fecal-oral route, fomites, respiratory aerosols, poorly chlorinated swimming pools; spread human to human
- pediatric respiratory tract infections—serotypes 1, 2, 5
- military→acute respiratory disease—serotypes 4, 7

Clinical Syndromes

1. Acute febrile pharyngitis: <3-year-old children; pharyngoconjunctival fever
2. Acute respiratory disease
3. Conjunctivitis: palpebral conjunctivitis nodular and both inflamed, hyperemia; eyes become crusted
4. Epidemic keratoconjunctivitis—hazard for workers in dust, foreign bodies, and other irritants: one eye becomes painful, red, watery, itchy, hyperemic, lid is swollen, ptosis, folliculitis, membranes or pseudomembranes
5. Gastroenteritis and diarrhea (serogroups 40, 41)
6. Bladder infection
7. Disseminated infection: meningitis, encephalitis, or hepatitis
8. Intussusception and congenital abnormalities

Immunity

- antibody→resolves lytic infection
- cell-mediated immunity→latent infections
  ⇒ limit viral outgrowth

Laboratory Diagnosis

- pharyngitis cases—must rule out *Streptococcus pyogenes*
- immunoassays include IFA on respiratory or conjunctival cells and EIA for adenovirus 40 and 41 on infant stools

Treatment

- no treatment
- immunization—serotype vaccine for 4 and 7 for military (→vacuum on lung)
- control with proper hygiene

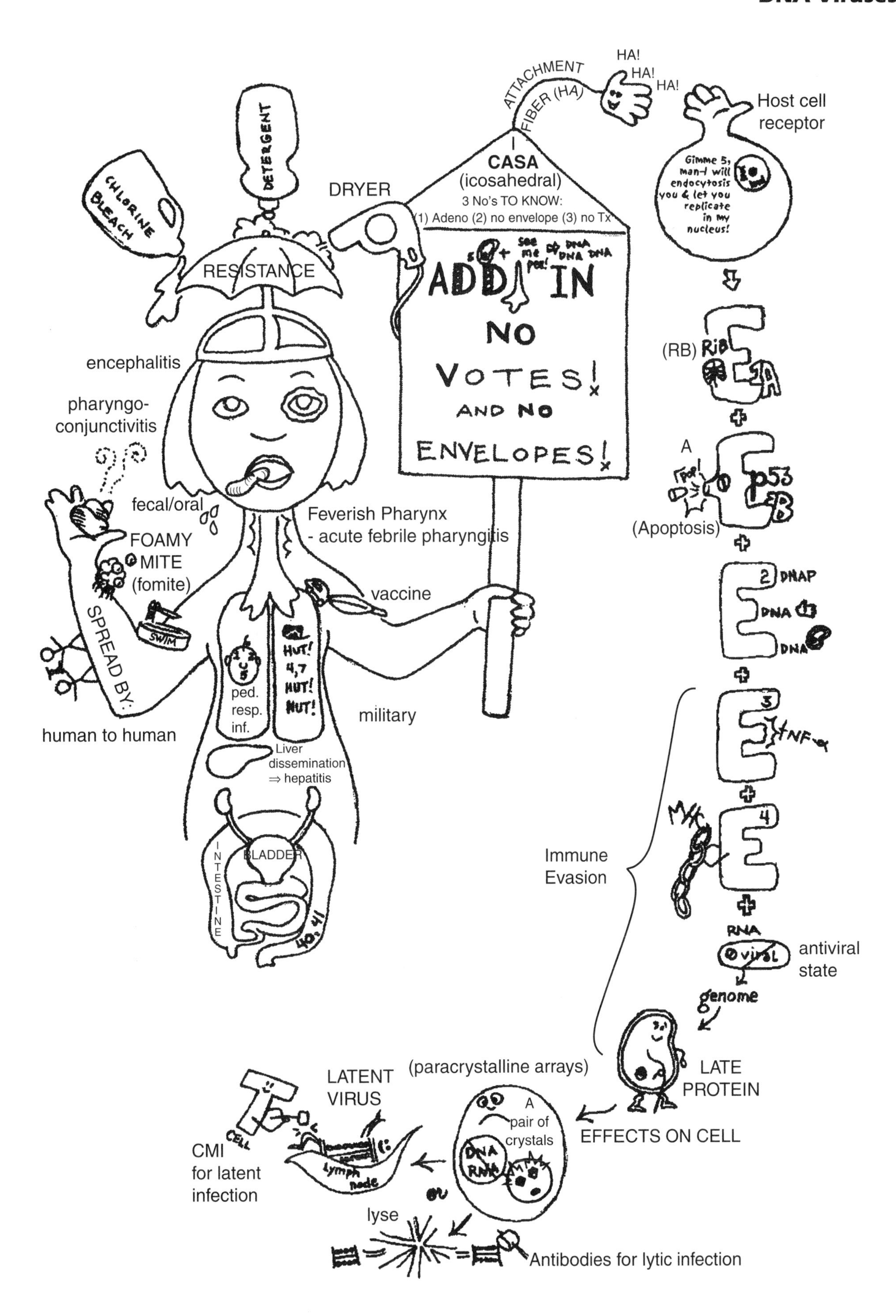
DETERGENT
CHLORINE BLEACH
RESISTANCE
DRYER
ATTACHMENT FIBER (HA)
HA!
HA!
HA!
Host cell receptor
Gimme 5, man-I will endocytosis you & let you replicate in my nucleus!
CASA
(icosahedral)
3 No's TO KNOW:
(1) Adeno (2) no envelope (3) no Tx
ADD IN
NO
VOTES!
AND NO
ENVELOPES!
encephalitis
pharyngo-conjunctivitis
fecal/oral
FOAMY MITE (fomite)
SWIM
SPREAD BY:
human to human
Feverish Pharynx
- acute febrile pharyngitis
vaccine
ped. resp. inf.
HUT! 4,7 HUT! HUT!
military
Liver dissemination ⇒ hepatitis
BLADDER
INTESTINE
40, 41
(RB)
A
p53
B
(Apoptosis)
2
DNAP
DNA
3
TNF-α
4
MHC
Immune Evasion
RNA
antiviral state
genome
LATE PROTEIN
EFFECTS ON CELL
(paracrystalline arrays)
A pair of crystals
DNA
RNA
LATENT VIRUS
CELL
CMI for latent infection
Lymph node
or
lyse
Antibodies for lytic infection

NOTES

PARVOVIRIDAE

DISEASE BIPHASIC

Initial Febrile Stage

- infectious stage; decreased hemoglobin
- nonspecific "flu" symptoms
- antibody developed
- viremia stops
- infection resolves
  - ⇒ stem cells will
- increase RBCs to replenish

Second Symptomatic Stage

- noninfectious
- symptom: rash, arthritis
- IgM Antibodies against parvovirus B=19
  - ⇒ binds viruses in immune complexes

Erythema (Biphasic) Infectiosum

- (1) and (2) refer to stages above
- 5th disease
  →(1) incubation→chills, etc.→3 days →↓ Hb→(2)→"slapped cheek" rash→spreads
- may reappear after bathing or sun exposure

Polyarthritis

- females, hands, wrists, knees

Immunocompromised

- ⇒ chronic anemia

Transient Aplastic Anemia

- most serious
- aplastic crisis
  ⇒↓Hb
- signs of heart failure may be present

Hydrops Fetalis

- Female catches P. B-19 when pregnant→virus crosses placenta during viremic phase
  - ⇒ occupational hazards for pregnant school teachers
- infant has generalized edema and ascites→hydrops fetalis
- hydrops fetalis and anemia together

Virus Types

- divided into two groups, both of which require additional factors for their replication:
  1. dependent—require proteins from other viruses (adeno or herpes) hard to replicate
  2. independent viruses require an actively replicating cell (S phase)
- small, non-enveloped, icosahedral
- linear ssDNA consisting of either + or – DNA strands→packaged separately at an approximately equal ratio
- genome encodes 5 proteins→1 promoter

Replicative Cycle

- only replicate in mitotically active cells; prefers to infect erythroid cell
  - ⇒ bone marrow and fetal liver erythroid
- binds to erythrocyte P-antigen (globoside)→internalized→uncoating→ ssDNA to nucleus→replicate in S phase + cellular DNAP→
  - ⇒ DNA replication primed by hairpin structures (formed by inverted repeats at either end of genome) and occurs by rolling hairpin mechanism→ alternate (+) and (–) strands are produced→ nicked for separation into individual genomes
- no temporal control of gene expression
- virions released cell lysis

Pathogenesis

- viremia peaks at 1 week and virus is shed from respiratory tract
- virus reaches the bone marrow where it multiplies in and destroys erythroid precursors→by day ten there are no erythroblasts in the bone marrow and no reticulocytes in the blood
- individuals with sickle cell, thalassemia, or hereditary spherocytosis have RBCs with lifespan of 15–20 days→they become anemic
- disease is biphasic

Epidemiology

- ubiquitous
- most common among 4–15 year olds
- occur in late winter and early spring
- transmission via respiratory aerosols and oral secretions and occurs easily as contagion precedes symptoms
- fomite spread can occur since virus environmentally stable→found viable after years of storage
- transmitted in blood products
- crosses the placenta; predilection for fetal erythroid cells

Diagnosis

- differentiate erythema infectiosum from rubella
  - ⇒ confirm cause of aplastic crisis or diagnose chronic disease
- definitive→demonstration of B-19 specific IgM or rising specific IgG titers

Treatment

none
- blood transfusion may be needed for aplastic anemia

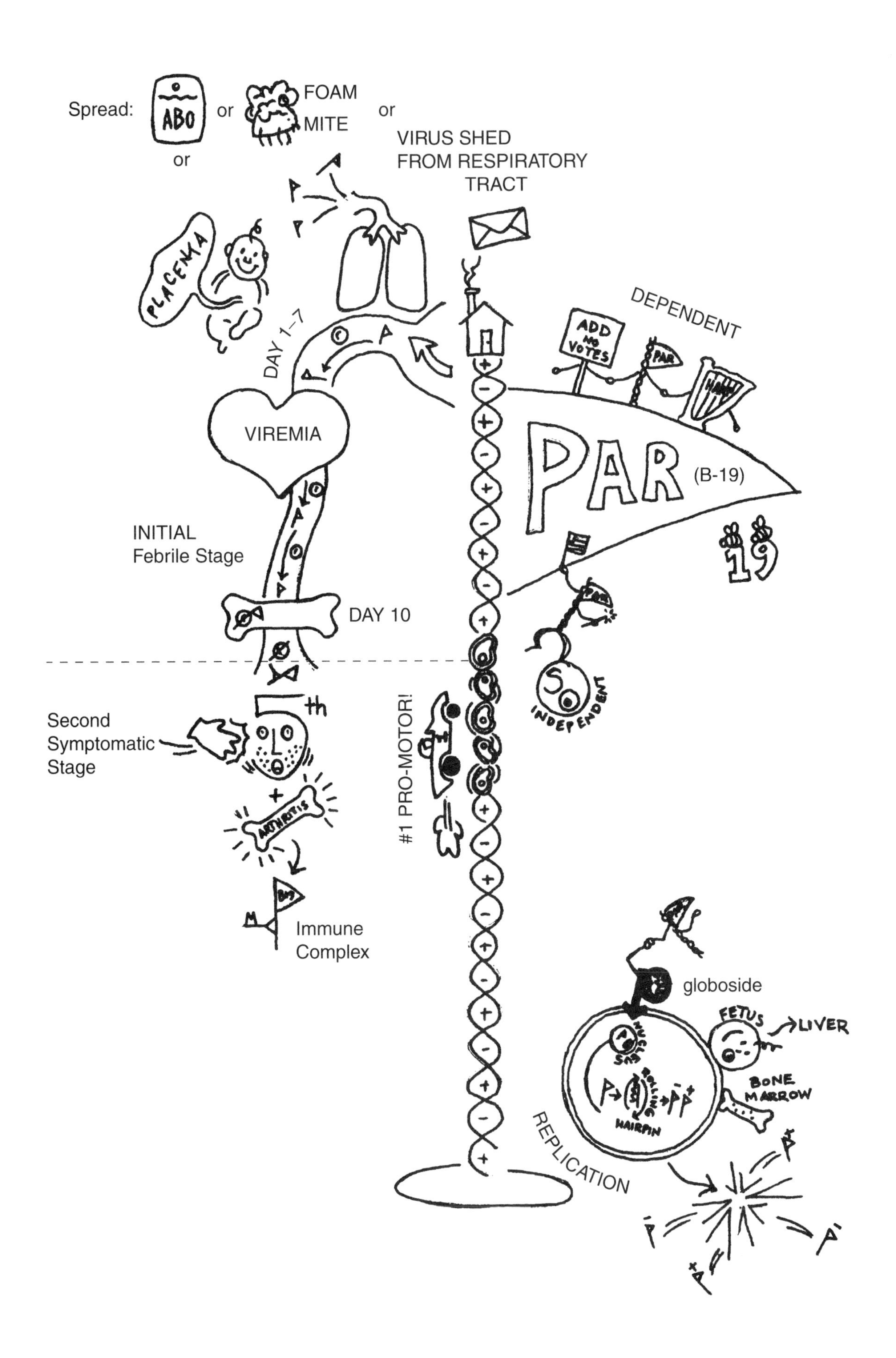
Spread:
ABO
or
FOAM
MITE
or
or
VIRUS SHED
FROM RESPIRATORY
TRACT
PLACENTA
DAY 1–7
VIREMIA
DEPENDENT
ADD NO VOTES
PAR
PAR
(B-19)
19
INITIAL
Febrile Stage
DAY 10
INDEPENDENT
Second
Symptomatic
Stage
5th
+
ARTHRITIS
#1 PRO-MOTOR!
Immune
Complex
globoside
FETUS
LIVER
BONE
MARROW
HAIRPIN
REPLICATION

PAPOVAVIRIDAE

PAPILLOMA

Pathogenesis

1. The virus first infects the basal cells of the stratum germinativum. Expression of early genes causes cells to hypertrophy. As cells mature, late viral proteins are synthesized and virions are produced. **The nucleus degenerates and a large vacuole develops (koilocytosis).** Viruses are shed when keratinocytes slough off.
2. Hypertrophy of the epithelium leads to acanthocytosis and development of a papilloma 3 months to 2 years after infection. The papilloma shows hyperkeratosis of the stratum corneum and stratum lucidum; **parakeratosis** of the stratum granulosum; acanthosis of the stratum spinorum (prickle cells) and the presence of koilocytes (virus-producing vacuolated cells).
3. **Spontaneous resolution occurs.** What triggers this is not known although **evidence suggests cell-mediated immunity.** Lymphocytic infiltration is present at this time and immunosuppressed persons have more recurrences and more serious infections.
4. Progression of an HPV infection to carcinoma occurs with types 16 and 18 (cervical), 6 (anogenital), and 5, 8, and 14 (squamous cell carcinoma from epidermodysplasia verruciformis). **It requires integration of the HPV genome into the host chromosome. This eliminates expression of viral E1 and E2 and allows full expression of E6 and E7 resulting in the loss of the suppressor protein p53 and tumor suppressor proteins RB and p107.** An environmental cofactor is also required. Smoking has been shown to increase the risk of progression to cancer.

- 6, 11: cervical dysplasia, laryngeal warts
  - ⇒ children are born with HPV
- genital warts
  - ⇒ condyloma accuminatum
  - ⇒ 16, 18

E1 = DNA binding protein for enhanced replication of the genome
E2 = transcriptional modulator
E6 = oncogenic, transforming: binds p53, speeding the rate at which p53 is degraded
E7 = oncogenic, transforming: binds retinoblastoma (RB) protein and p107
L1 = major capsid protein
L2 = minor capsid protein

Epidemiology

1. The major means of transmission is **person to person by direct contact.** Acquisition occurs through breaks in the skin or mucous membranes. Inoculation can also occur during sexual intercourse or passage through an infected birth canal.
2. HPV can be transmitted on **fomites (bathroom floors or towels) because it resists in activation; medical instruments must be steam sterilized.**

Treatment

surgical excision, cryotherapy, salicylic and lactic acid paint, 10% glutaraldehyde + 5-fluorouracil or podophyllum resin

POLYOMAVIRUS

Structure and Replication

- human polyomaviruses (BK and JC virus)
- dsDNA genome: 3 regions

1) Early
   - large T protein: uses ATP, acts as helicase, binds DNA to control early and late gene transcription and DNA replication, surface glycoprotein, oncogene, binds and inactivates p53 and RB→stimulates cell from G_o to S phase
   - middle T: oncogenic
   - small t: cell transformation
2) Noncoding region: contains origin of replication and the star sequence for transcriptional regulation of both early and late genes
3) Late genes: produce capsid proteins
   - outcome: permissive cells→cell lysis after replication; nonpermissive→viral genome integrates resulting in transformation of the cell and no virion production

Pathogenesis

1° infection usually asymptomatic
JC and BK→enter via respiratory tract→

BK	JC
↓	↓
establishes in kidney	establishes in kidney, B-cells, and monocytic cells
↓	↓
immunocompromised (virus reactivates and sheds)	
↓	↓
BK: severe urinary infection in kidney transplant patients and bone marrow patients→see pictures	JC: viremia and CNS infection ⇒ crosses blood–brain barrier in endothelial cells→ (1) **abortive infection** of astrocytes→ enlarged glioblastoma-like cells (2) productive infection→(lytic) of oligodendrocytes causes demyelination →PML (progressive multifocal leukoencephalopathy)→ in immunocompromised; defined by neurologic symptoms indicating multiple lesions→ CNS effects: aphasia, ataxia, etc. followed by dementia, coma, death within 10 months

Diagnosis

histological findings **brain tissue ⇒lesions within the white matter consisting** of asymmetric foci of demyelination surrounded by oligodendrocytes containing inclusions are characteristic of the disease→ enlarged cells with dense basophilic intranuclear inclusions similar to CMV inclusions but larger without owl's eye halo

Treatment

cytosine arabinoside, IFN-α, idoxuridine, zidovudine

NOTES

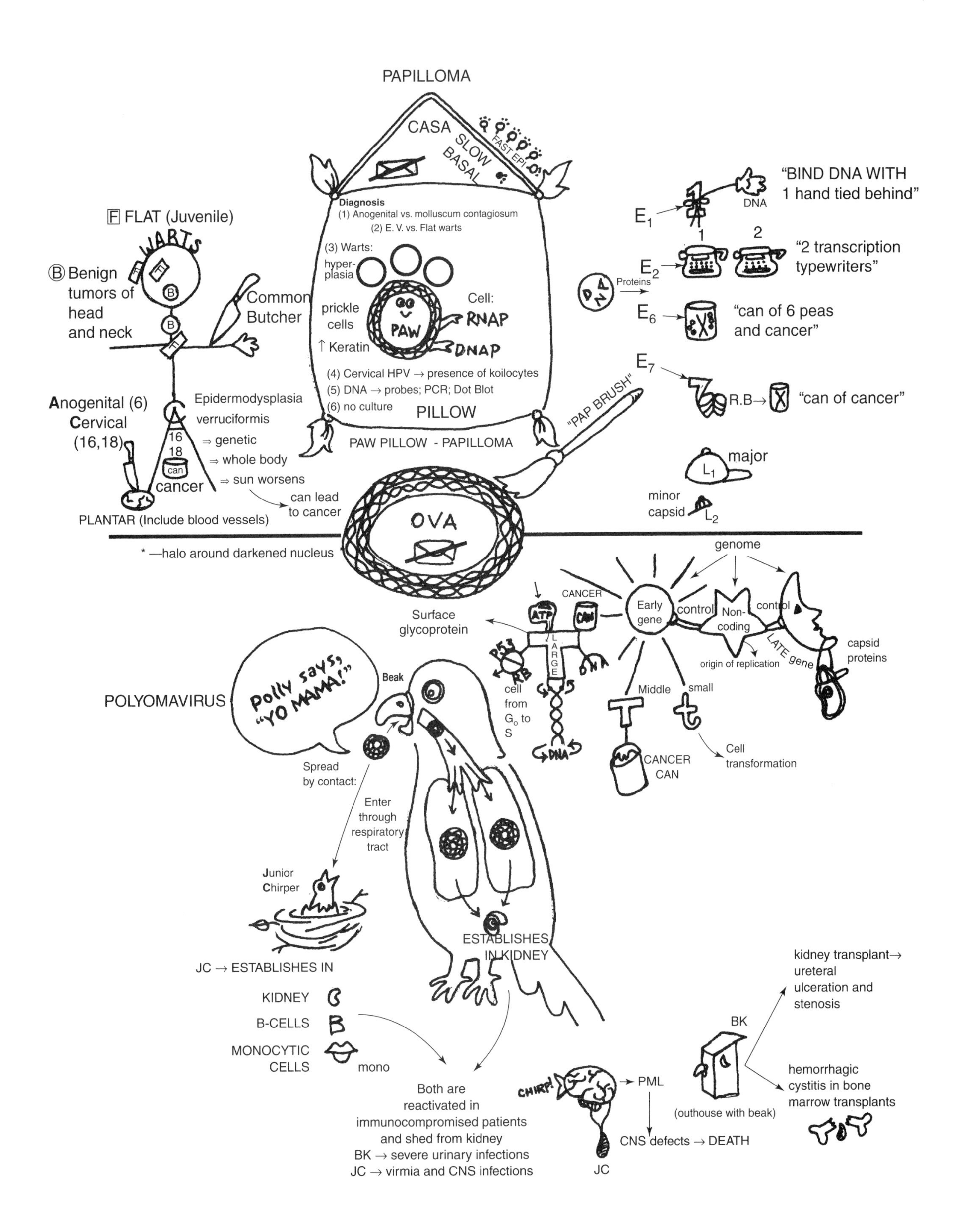
PAPILLOMA
CASA
SLOW
BASAL
FAST EPI
Diagnosis
(1) Anogenital vs. molluscum contagiosum
(2) E. V. vs. Flat warts
(3) Warts:
hyper-plasia
prickle cells
↑ Keratin
PAW
Cell:
RNAP
DNAP
(4) Cervical HPV → presence of koilocytes
(5) DNA → probes; PCR; Dot Blot
(6) no culture
PILLOW
PAW PILLOW - PAPILLOMA
F FLAT (Juvenile)
WARTS
B Benign tumors of head and neck
Common Butcher
Anogenital (6)
Cervical (16,18)
16
18
can
cancer
Epidermodysplasia verruciformis
⇒ genetic
⇒ whole body
⇒ sun worsens
can lead to cancer
PLANTAR (Include blood vessels)
* —halo around darkened nucleus
OVA
"PAP BRUSH"
E1
DNA
"BIND DNA WITH 1 hand tied behind"
1
2
E2
Proteins
"2 transcription typewriters"
E6
"can of 6 peas and cancer"
E7
R.B→
"can of cancer"
major
L1
minor capsid
L2
genome
CANCER
ATP
CAN
Early gene
control
Non-coding
control
origin of replication
LATE gene
capsid proteins
Surface glycoprotein
P53
RB
LARGE
DNA
cell from G0 to S
Middle
small
CANCER CAN
Cell transformation
POLYOMAVIRUS
Polly says, "YO MAMA!"
Beak
Spread by contact:
Enter through respiratory tract
Junior Chirper
ESTABLISHES IN KIDNEY
JC → ESTABLISHES IN
KIDNEY
B-CELLS
MONOCYTIC CELLS
mono
Both are reactivated in immunocompromised patients and shed from kidney
BK → severe urinary infections
JC → virmia and CNS infections
CHIRP!
→ PML
CNS defects → DEATH
JC
BK
(outhouse with beak)
kidney transplant→ ureteral ulceration and stenosis
hemorrhagic cystitis in bone marrow transplants

NOTES

HERPESVIRIDAE

⇒ "harp"

Structure

- genome associated with toroidal core protein; enclosed in icosadeltahedral capsid; capsid surrounded by amorphous protein tegument and enclosed in a glycoprotein-studded envelope forming large spherical virions
- because of envelope→sensitive to acid detergents, drying, and organic solvents
- linear dsDNA genome contains reiterated sequences that bracket the unique long (U_L) and unique short (U_S) sequences→ these repeat regions allow circularization and recombination of the genome→which switches the orientation of U_L and U_S
- second largest viruses known

Replication

interaction of viral attachment proteins with cell surface receptors→**(tropism restricted by tissue specific expression of particular CSR)**→virus enters cell by viropexis→ nucleocapsid uncoated at nuclear pores→viral genome enters nucleus→transcription and protein synthesis occur in 3 phases→interaction determines outcome (lytic, persistent, latent)

Proteins

immediate early (α) proteins: transcription regulated by α transduction factor that is carried into nucleus along with the genome→α-transcripts encode phosphorylases that transactivate β-genes
delayed early (β) proteins: inactivate α-genes; include thymidine kinase, DNAP, DNA-binding proteins for replication; transcriptional factors that turn on γ genes

Temporal Control

late proteins: structural

- genome replicated by viral DNAP
- envelope acquired at nuclear membrane
- release: exocytosis or cell lysis
- **control replication**
- **establish latent infection in neurons**
- initial infection is epithelial and mucosal

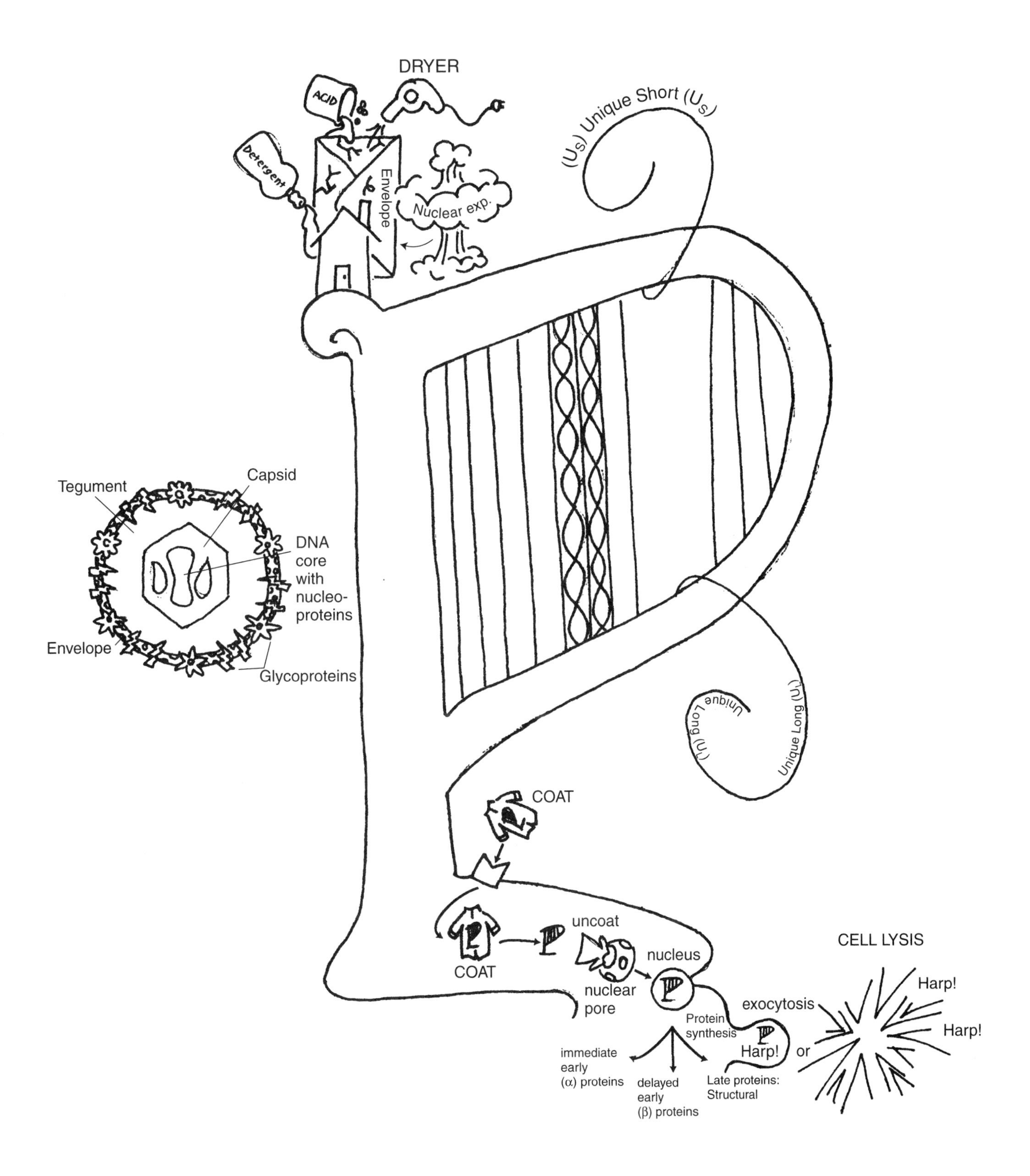
DRYER
ACID
Detergent
Envelope
Nuclear exp.
(Us) Unique Short (Us)
Tegument
Capsid
DNA
core
with
nucleo-
proteins
Envelope
Glycoproteins
Unique Long (UL)
Long (UL)
Unique
COAT
COAT
uncoat
nucleus
nuclear
pore
exocytosis
Protein
synthesis
Harp!
or
CELL LYSIS
Harp!
Harp!
immediate
early
(α) proteins
delayed
early
(β) proteins
Late proteins:
Structural

HERPES SIMPLEX

Pathogenesis

1. Virus attaches to heparan sulfate on cell surface and then attaches to another cell surface receptor.
2. Lytic infections involve the epithelial cells and fibroblast cells, specifically, in the parabasal and intermediate epithelial cells at the site of entry.
3. Syncytia form with Cowdry-type intranuclear inclusions.
4. Nucleus becomes engorged and cell lysis occurs.
5. Resolution of the infection requires CMI (cell-mediated immunity).
6. Cytotoxic lymphocytes (CTLs) produce antiviral cytokines which induce latent infection.
7. The virus enters sensory neurons and travels to the dorsal root ganglion (DRG) via retrograde intra-axonal transport. (HSV-1 to the trigeminal DRG; HSV-2 to the sacral DRG.)
8. During the latency period α-genes are repressed and latency associated transcripts (nonsense RNA) bind up viral transcripts and inhibit protein translation.
9. Upon reactivation the virus returns to the initial site of infection via the neuron.

Epidemiology

- HSV-1 can be differentiated from HSV-2 by its growth at 40°C
- both can infect the same tissues: mucoepithelial cells and skin tissue where breaks are present
- no animal reservoirs or vectors
- contracted by direct contact with secretions: HSV-1 by oral contact during childhood and during contact sports; HSV-2 by sexual contact where primary infections occur after puberty
- mother can transmit to fetus: transmission to fetus more likely if mother's infection is primary instead of recurrent because in a primary infection the mother will not have antibodies to also transmit to fetus; scalp electrodes also increase likelihood of transmission to fetus

Clinical Syndromes

Primary Infections with HSV-1

- **gingivostomatitis:** common in those less than 5 years old; lesion throughout mouth; primarily stays in epithelial layer—no viremia; virus latent in trigeminal root ganglion
- **herpetic pharyngitis** without gingivostomatitis; infection in those more than 5 years old
- **follicular conjunctivitis** or **blepharitis** (lesions in eye margins)
- **skin infections: herpetic whitlow**—involves 1 finger with itching and pain; **herpes gladiatorum**—skin infections on various body parts of those who play contact sports

Primary Infections with HSV-2

- **genital herpes:** via sexual contact; may experience meningitis; virus latent in lumbar DRG

Recurrent Infections

- **herpes labialis:** cold sores and fever blisters; prodrome of itching and burning prior to appearance of vesicles
- **herpetic keratitis** (attacks cornea) or keratoconjunctivitis: ulcers may cause blindness
- **recurrent genital herpes:** virus is shed even after healing

Complications of HSV

- **congenital infection**
- **HSV encephalitis:** most common cause of sporadic encephalitis; spreads to brain via the neuronal route during a primary infection or recurrence; usually caused by HSV-1; infection produces necrotizing hemorrhagic encephalitis in one of the temporal lobes; high fatality rate and those who survive over 90% have permanent neurological damage

Infections of the immunocompromised

- **eczema herpeticum:** HSV spreads through existing eczema
- **visceral or disseminated HSV**

Laboratory Diagnosis

- **direct:** examine scrapings from lesions looking for multinucleated giants cells; **use rapid immunofluorescent assay**
- **viral culture, serology** to determine immune status or if this was a primary or recurrent (HSV-specific IgM) infection
- **molecular diagnosis:** PCR detects virus DNA in CNS or tears

Prevention and Treatment

- **acyclovir** used for active infection; **foscarnet** can be used if resistance develops; **vidarabine** treats encephalitis or neonatal HSV infection; prevention is best by avoiding contact with lesions

SIMIAN HERPESVIRUS B

Epidemiology

- natural pathogen of rhesus and cynomolgus monkeys; human becomes infected from contact with oral or genital secretions

Clinical Syndrome

- lesions appear at site of entry and progressive ascending myelitis follows; followed by severe headache, fever, hemorrhagic encephalitis, etc.; infection is usually fatal

Laboratory Diagnosis

virus is Biosafety Level 4 Pathogen

Treatment

acyclovir or ganciclovir when infection is local; wound should be washed immediately with bleach or iodine

VARICELLA-ZOSTER VIRUS (VZV)

Structure and Replication

- smallest genome; only enveloped virions are infectious; replicates more slowly than HSV; latent infection in neurons

Pathogenesis

- primary replication site is respiratory tract where it multiplies rapidly→spreads via bloodstream and lymphatics to the RES and multiplies again→secondary viremia→spreads virus throughout the body→replicates in monocytes, capillary endothelial cells, and epithelial cells→rash erupts
- rash is dermal vesiculopustular that involves the corium and dermis; contains polynucleated giant cells with ballooning degeneration and eosinophilic intranuclear inclusions
- virus-specific CTLs stimulate virus to enter sensory nerve and travel to DRG; reactivates in those with impaired CMI; when reactivated a vesicular rash erupts in the dermatome fed by the nerve

Epidemiology

- **chickenpox (varicella)** is endemic; once infected with varicella can develop shingles (herpes zoster) with incidence increasing with age or immunosuppression
- highly contagious; spread by respiratory droplets during prodrome and by contact; contagion precedes symptoms by 48 hours and continues until all lesions are crusted
- **shingles**—lesions can spread varicella to susceptible individual who will contract chickenpox

Clinical Syndromes

- **chickenpox**—incubation period of 2–3 weeks, fever occurs and rash erupts; begins as a small macule→to clear vesicle on a maculopapular base→to vesicle that becomes pustular and then crusted→ spreads centrifugally over the body; lesions itch intensely but scratching can lead to bacterial infection; mucous membrane lesions can appear on conjunctiva, mouth, and vagina

Complications

cerebellar ataxia, **encephalitis, Guillain-Barré or Reye's syndrome, hemorrhagic or visceral infection, congenital infection**

Reactivation Infection

shingles—follows nerve to dermatome; intense neuritis prior to rash; usually one-sided; **postherpetic neuralgia; ophthalmia**

Laboratory Diagnosis

diagnosis clinically; identified with immunofluorescent assays; serology screens for immunity

Treatment

life-threatening infection→**IV acyclovir; oral acyclovir** speeds healing of shingles; protection after infection is life-long; vaccine (live)

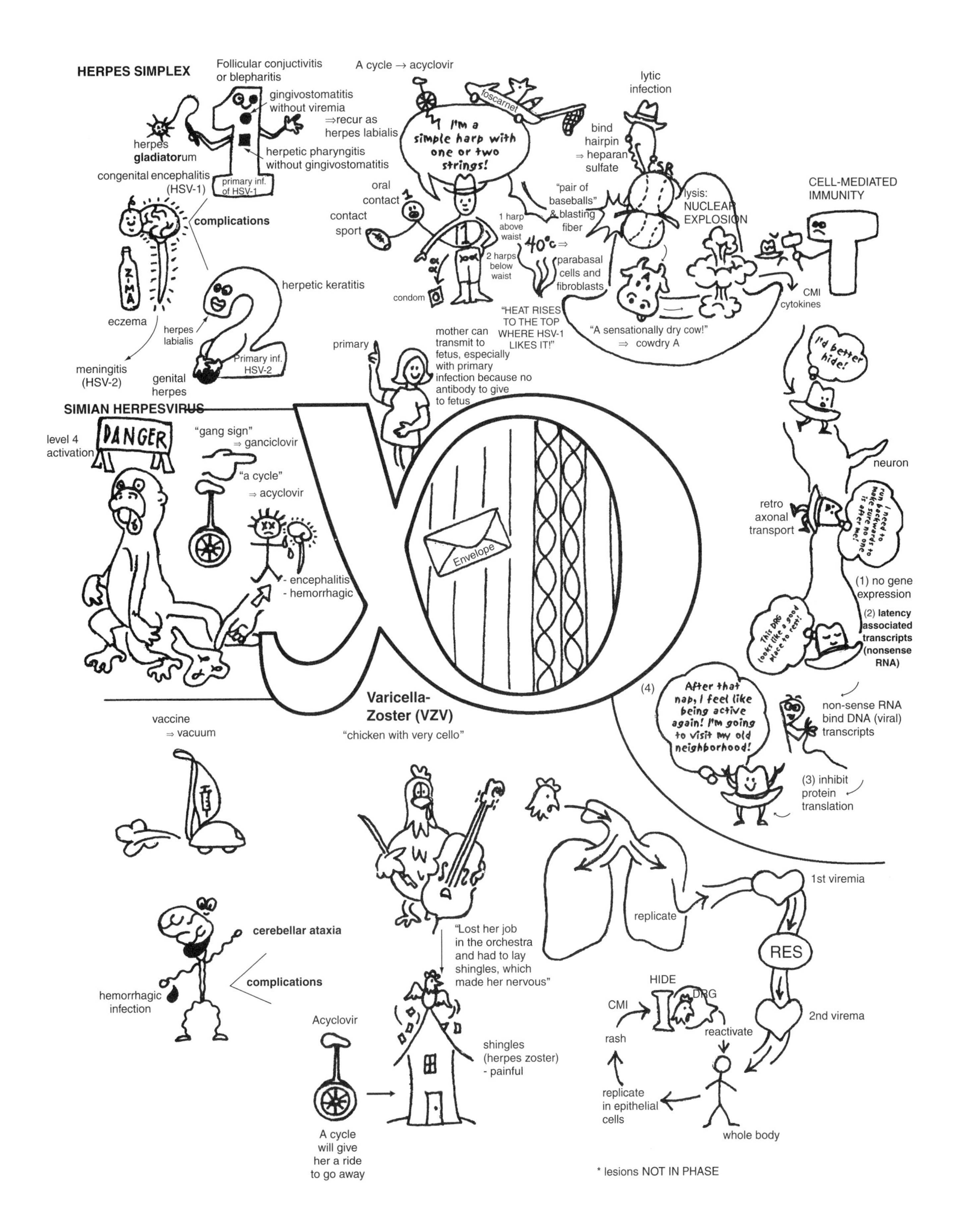
HERPES SIMPLEX
Follicular conjuctivitis or blepharitis
gingivostomatitis without viremia
⇒recur as herpes labialis
herpetic pharyngitis without gingivostomatitis
herpes gladiatorum
congenital encephalitis (HSV-1)
primary inf. of HSV-1
complications
ZIMA
eczema
herpetic keratitis
herpes labialis
Primary inf. HSV-2
meningitis (HSV-2)
genital herpes
A cycle → acyclovir
foscarnet
I'm a simple harp with one or two strings!
oral contact
contact sport
1 harp above waist
2 harps below waist
condom
40°c ⇒
parabasal cells and fibroblasts
"HEAT RISES TO THE TOP WHERE HSV-1 LIKES IT!"
lytic infection
bind hairpin ⇒ heparan sulfate
"pair of baseballs" & blasting fiber
lysis: NUCLEAR EXPLOSION
"A sensationally dry cow!" ⇒ cowdry A
CELL-MEDIATED IMMUNITY
CMI cytokines
primary
mother can transmit to fetus, especially with primary infection because no antibody to give to fetus
I'd better hide!
neuron
retro axonal transport
I need to run backwards to make sure no one is after me!
(1) no gene expression
(2) latency associated transcripts (nonsense RNA)
This DRG looks like a good place to rest!
SIMIAN HERPESVIRUS
DANGER
level 4 activation
"gang sign" ⇒ ganciclovir
"a cycle" ⇒ acyclovir
- encephalitis
- hemorrhagic
Envelope
Varicella-Zoster (VZV)
"chicken with very cello"
(4)
After that nap, I feel like being active again! I'm going to visit my old neighborhood!
non-sense RNA bind DNA (viral) transcripts
(3) inhibit protein translation
vaccine ⇒ vacuum
cerebellar ataxia
complications
hemorrhagic infection
"Lost her job in the orchestra and had to lay shingles, which made her nervous"
shingles (herpes zoster) - painful
Acyclovir
A cycle will give her a ride to go away
replicate
1st viremia
RES
2nd virema
HIDE
DRG
CMI
rash
reactivate
replicate in epithelial cells
whole body
* lesions NOT IN PHASE

NOTES

BETA HERPESVIRIDAE

⇒ slow, non-lytic

CYTOMEGALOVIRUS (CMV)

Structure and Replication

- large and enveloped; replicates only in human cells; permissive cells→fibroblasts, epithelial cells and macrophages; latent infection in lymphocytes, bone marrow stromal cells, kidney cells, and ductal cells

Pathogenesis and Immunity

- infections are generally asymptomatic except in immunocompromised patients; can lie dormant for years; infection considered life long; CMI required for infection resolution; natural killer cells provide early protection
- CMV evades immune response by moving directly from cell to cell; reduces cellular expression of MHC class I antigen by substituting its own UL18 protein for the heavy chain of MHC class I; free virions accumulate a coat of β2-microglobulin; CMV envelope protein serves as an Fc receptor for antibodies

Epidemiology

- transmitted by most body fluids
- source of infection varies with age: neonate—transplacental or intrauterine; cervical secretions during birth; infant/child—breast milk, saliva, tears, urine; adult—sexual transmission, blood transfusion, organ transplants (most severe in bone marrow transplants who develop interstitial pneumonia) major cause of death among AIDS patients

Clinical Syndromes

- **congenital CMV—leading cause of congenital birth defects;** cytomegalic inclusion disease—infant stillborn; **deafness** and visual impairment
- **perinatal CMV**—usually asymptomatic
- **infection in children and adults: asymptomatic; heterophile-negative mononucleosis:** pharyngitis, lymphadenopathy, hepatitis, atypical lymphocytes but no heterophile antibody; complications include Guillain–Barré, myocarditis, thrombocytopenia, hemolytic anemia
- **transfusion-acquired CMV:** appears as mononucleosis
- **organ transplant acquired** can be life-threatening; graft rejection
- **AIDS patients:** develop chorioretinitis, encephalitis, colitis/esophagitis

Laboratory Diagnosis

- histology—finding of owl's eye cells in tissue is pathognomonic

Treatment

- ganciclovir and foscarnet; no vaccine available

HUMAN HERPESVIRUSES 6 AND 7 (HHV-6 AND HHV-7)

- primary tropism for CD4+ T-cells; remain latent in macrophages and salivary gland cells; HHV-6—adults; HHV-7—febrile children

Epidemiology

- **both spread via saliva**

Clinical Syndromes

- adults asymptomatic
- children: sudden fever, rash suddenly appears→roseola infantum

Laboratory Diagnosis

- clinical diagnosis, serologic demonstration of specific IgM or a 4-fold increase in specific IgG

Treatment

- ganciclovir and foscarnet

Beta Herpeviridae

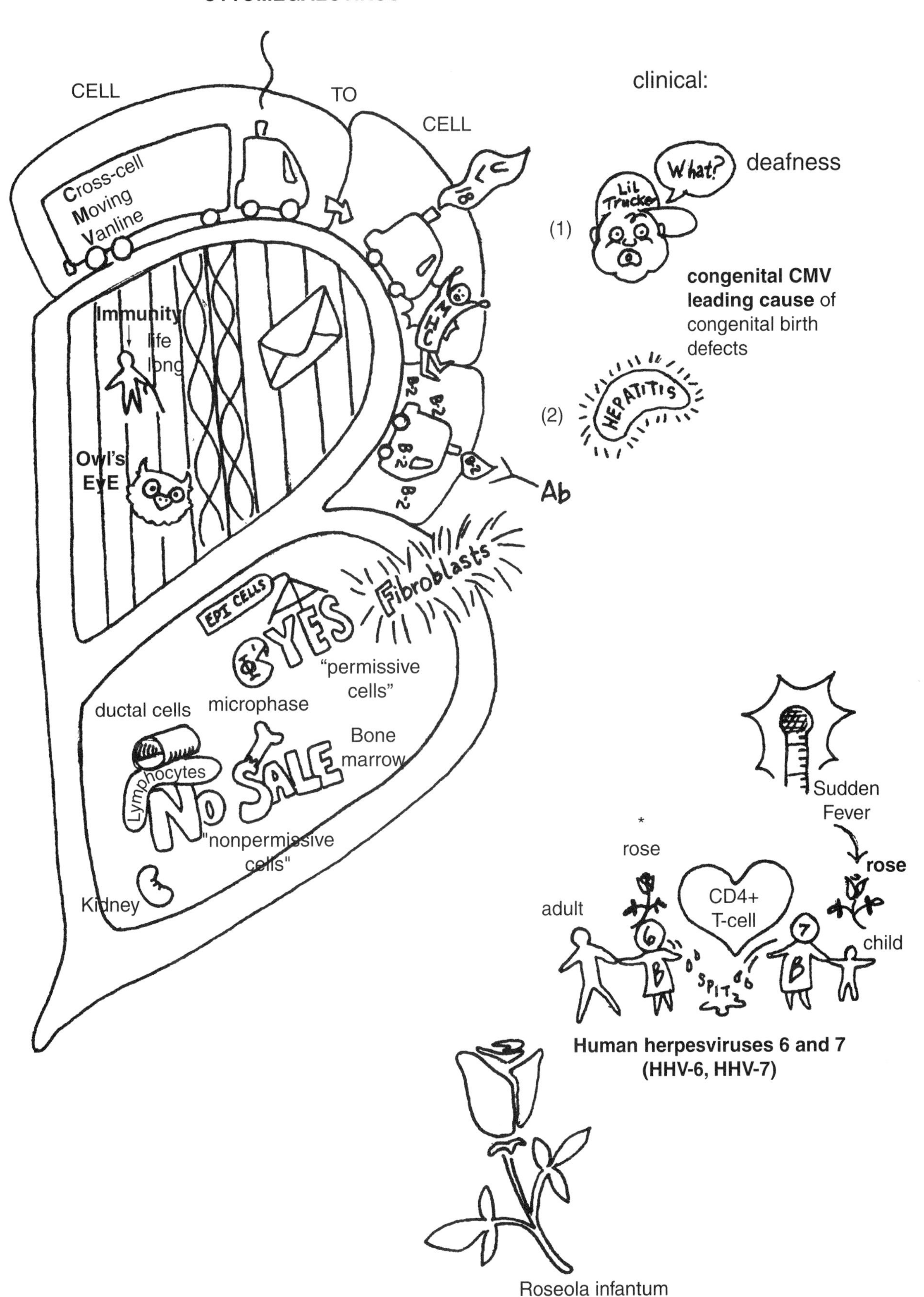

NOTES

EPSTEIN-BARR VIRUS (EBV)

Structure and Replication

- most prevalent of human viruses; syndrome of fever and lymphadenopathy with infectious mononucleosis
- two types: EBV-A found in B-cells of immunocompetent individuals; EBV-B found in B-cells from immunocompromised individuals
- EBV gp350/200 binds the Cd3 (CR2 or CD21) complement receptor for entry into cells **(this marker expressed only on B-cells and epithelial cells of the oropharynx and nasopharynx)**

Pathogenesis and Immunity

- infection of oropharyngeal epithelial cells→ followed by shedding of virus in saliva and entry of EBV into the B-cells of underlying lymphoid tissue→after second round of replication→disseminates to RES
- latent EBV infection alters the action of B-cells
- EBV genome as episome: only certain immediate early genes expressed (EB nuclear antigens→EBNAs, latent proteins, latent membrane proteins) and 2 small encoded EBV encoded RNAs (EBER-1 and EBER-2); **EBNA-1 binds and activates EBNA-2→immortalizes the cell**; B-cell growth factor is enhanced and the B-cell makes monoclonal IgM antibody (heterophile antibodies)
- immune response begins with antibodies against EBNAs and viral capsid antigens (VCA); CMI is primarily CD8+ T-cells that react to LMP-1 and EBNA-2 through 6→ CTLs destroy infected B-cells→controlling replication of the virus; **proliferating T-cells (appear as atypical or reactive lymphocytes) are known as Downey cells→without T-cell reaction→B-cells continue to proliferate and B-cell lymphoma occurs**
- **immune escape: EBV encodes an analog of IL-10 which inhibits the Th1 response**

Epidemiology

- transmitted in saliva during intimate contact or by sharing of eating and drinking utensils; virus shed for 18 months

Clinical Syndromes

- **infectious mononucleosis:** retro-orbital headache, feeling of abdominal fullness→ then lymphadenopathy and sore throat; grayish white exudates; if ampicillin given will develop rash
- complications: autoimmune hemolytic anemia, splenic rupture, Guillain-Barré syndrome, encephalitis
- **chronic EBV infection: NOT chronic fatigue syndrome**
- immunosuppressed: develop polyclonal lymphoma or monoclonal B-cell lymphoma; AIDS patients—**hairy** oral leukoplakia
- **African Burkitt's lymphoma: monoclonal lymphoma of the jaw and face;** tumor cells contain a chromosomal translocation that brings the c-myc oncogene (chromosome 8) onto a chromosome carrying Ig genes (chromosome 2, 14, or 22); **joint with malarial infection**
- **nasopharyngeal carcinoma-tumor** cells (epithelial in origin); only EBNA-1 expressed; genetic marker possible in role of carcinoma; **(Asians)**

Laboratory Diagnosis

- lymphocytosis: atypical lymphocytes, larger than normal with curled edge, vacuolated cytoplasm, and basophilic lobulated eccentric nucleus
- heterophile antibodies; EBV specific antibodies

Treatment

- no treatment and no vaccine

HUMAN HERPESVIRUS 8

- detected by PCR isolation of DNA sequences from cells in Kaposi's sarcoma lesions and a rare type of B-cell lymphoma from AIDS patients; probably spread by intercourse

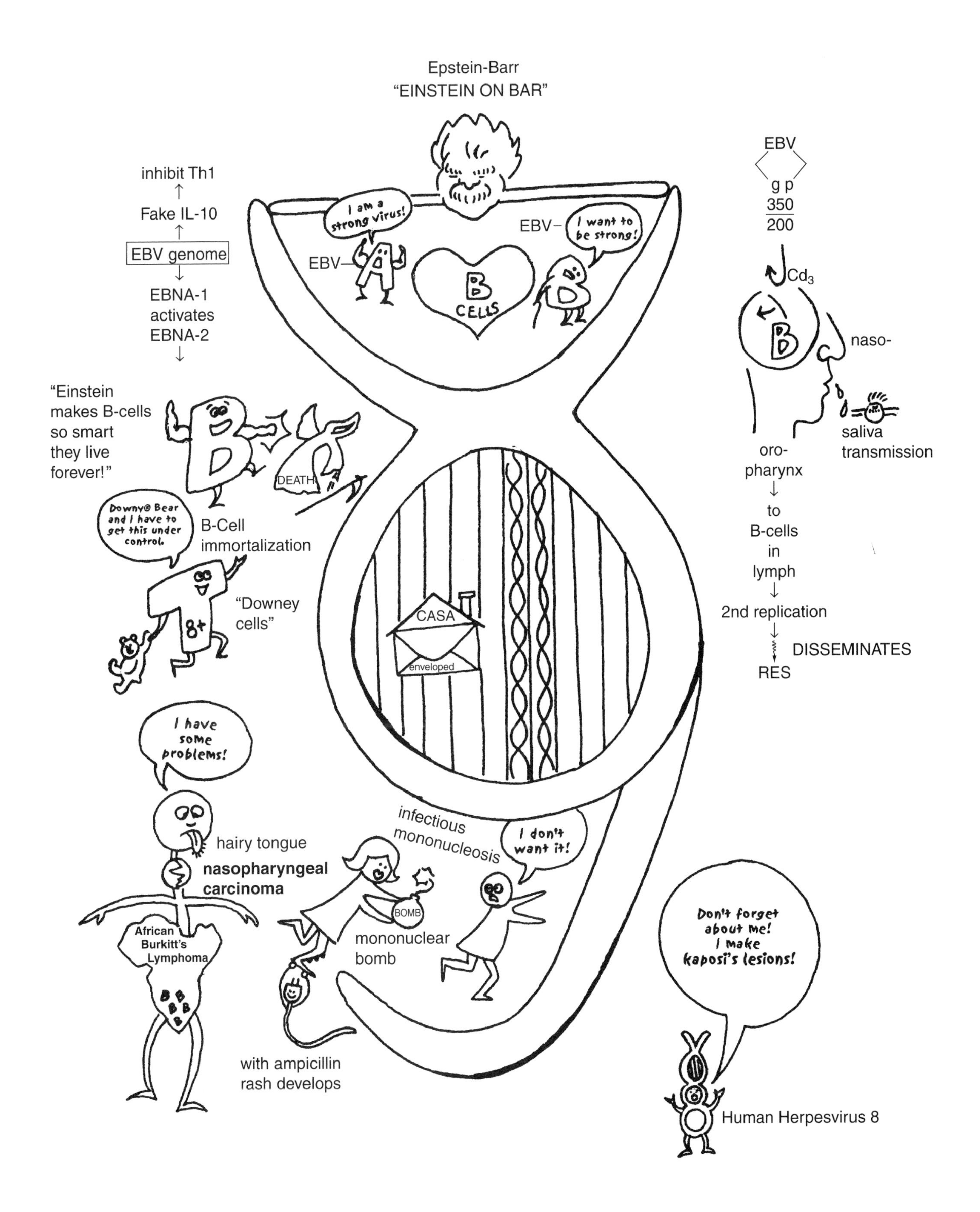
Epstein-Barr
"EINSTEIN ON BAR"
I am a strong virus!
EBV–
EBV–
I want to be strong!
B CELLS
inhibit Th1
Fake IL-10
EBV genome
EBNA-1
activates
EBNA-2
"Einstein makes B-cells so smart they live forever!"
DEATH
Downy® Bear and I have to get this under control.
B-Cell immortalization
8+
"Downey cells"
CASA
enveloped
EBV
g p
350
200
Cd3
B
naso-
saliva transmission
oro-pharynx
to
B-cells
in
lymph
2nd replication
DISSEMINATES
RES
I have some problems!
hairy tongue
nasopharyngeal carcinoma
African Burkitt's Lymphoma
infectious mononucleosis
I don't want it!
BOMB
mononuclear bomb
with ampicillin rash develops
Don't forget about me! I make kaposi's lesions!
Human Herpesvirus 8

POXVIRIDAE

"pox the box"

POXVIRIDAE

Structure and Replication

- strands of DNA linked covalently at or near termini; virion uncoated in two-stage process and the immediate early genes are read while the genome is still within the nucleocapsid core

NOTES

- **ONLY DNA VIRUS THAT REPLICATES IN CYTOPLASM**
- largest and most complex virus **known**—must carry with it everything
- pox virus→variola caused smallpox

Complex Structure

- brick-shaped virions, linear dsDNA
- replication takes place in cytoplasmic factories→visible as **acidophilic Guarnieri's bodies;** aggregates of mature virions accumulate as eosinophilic inclusions

Replication

- virus enters cell via membrane fusion→uncoating→first transcripts made while virion is in core→one of first products (uncoating enzyme) removes core membrane releasing genome into cell cytoplasm→delayed early genes transcribed (producing factors for DNA replication)→DNA replication semi-conservative and bidirectional→viral endonuclease cleaves lariat-shaped DNA progeny (templates for transcription of intermediate and late genes)→virions are assembled→released individually via cellular villi→post-translational processing of proteins by glycosylation, phosphorylation, or proteolytic cleavage is required for assembly→process inhibited by rifampicin→therefore, poxviruses are the ONLY VIRUSES SENSITIVE TO AN ANTIBACTERIAL AGENT

ORTHOPOXVIRUS

Epidemiology

- variola major→severe smallpox
- variola minor→alastrim
- vaccinia: originally attenuated cowpox; currently being studied for use in immunization of multiple diseases
- **smallpox (variola major and minor); transmitted via respiratory secretions; virus survived in scabs of pustules for months;** after fever came maculopapular rash on face, hands, forearms then to trunk and legs; after scabbing of lesions→cabs fall off and leave deep pockmarks (often disfiguring); no treatment
- 1980: WHO declared smallpox eradicated from the world which was possible because:
- **strictly human virus and only one serotype**
- **no asymptomatic carriers**
- high secondary attack rate
- everyone could be protected by smallpox vaccine

Vaccinia

- scarification, injection, or airjet administration; heals leaving pockmark

Complications

- encephalitis
- vaccinia gangrenosa—patient develops metastatic necrotic lesions, usually fatal
- eczema vaccinatum—individual with atopic dermatitis develop Kaposi's varicelliform eruption (can be treated with vaccinia Ig)
- generalized vaccinia <1 year old; numerous vesicles with bright red bases appear all over body; benign

Cowpox

- localized ulcerating lesions on hand and maybe also eye (from autoinoculation)

Buffalopox

- localized pustular lesions on hand

Monkeypox

- generalized eruption similar to smallpox

PARAPOXVIRUS

Milker's Nodule

- paravaccinia or pseudocowpox
- red papule develops 5–7 days after contact with lesion on the udder of infected cow
- **virus does not protect against smallpox**

Orf

- contagious pustular dermatitis or ecthyma contagiosum
- **transmitted from infected sheep or goats;** fomite transmission also possible
- papular erythematous lesion with red center surrounded by a white ring within area of inflammation

MOLLUSCIPOXVIRUS

- unique because noncultivatable in chicken egg chorioallantoic membranes or cell culture
- humans only host; virus transmitted by direct contact (often sexual) with lesions or on fomites such as towels and washcloths
- **molluscum contagiosum**—low-grade infection without mortality; **pearly papules; found anywhere on body except palms of hands and soles of feet**
- microscopic exam: hypertrophied and hyperplastic epithelium; molluscum bodies; cytoplasmic inclusions
- lesions heal spontaneously

YABAPOXVIRUS

Yabapoxvirus: transmitted to people who handle monkeys; characterized by development of a histiocytoma
Tanapoxvirus: disseminated by arthropod; single umbilicated papule forms at site of bite

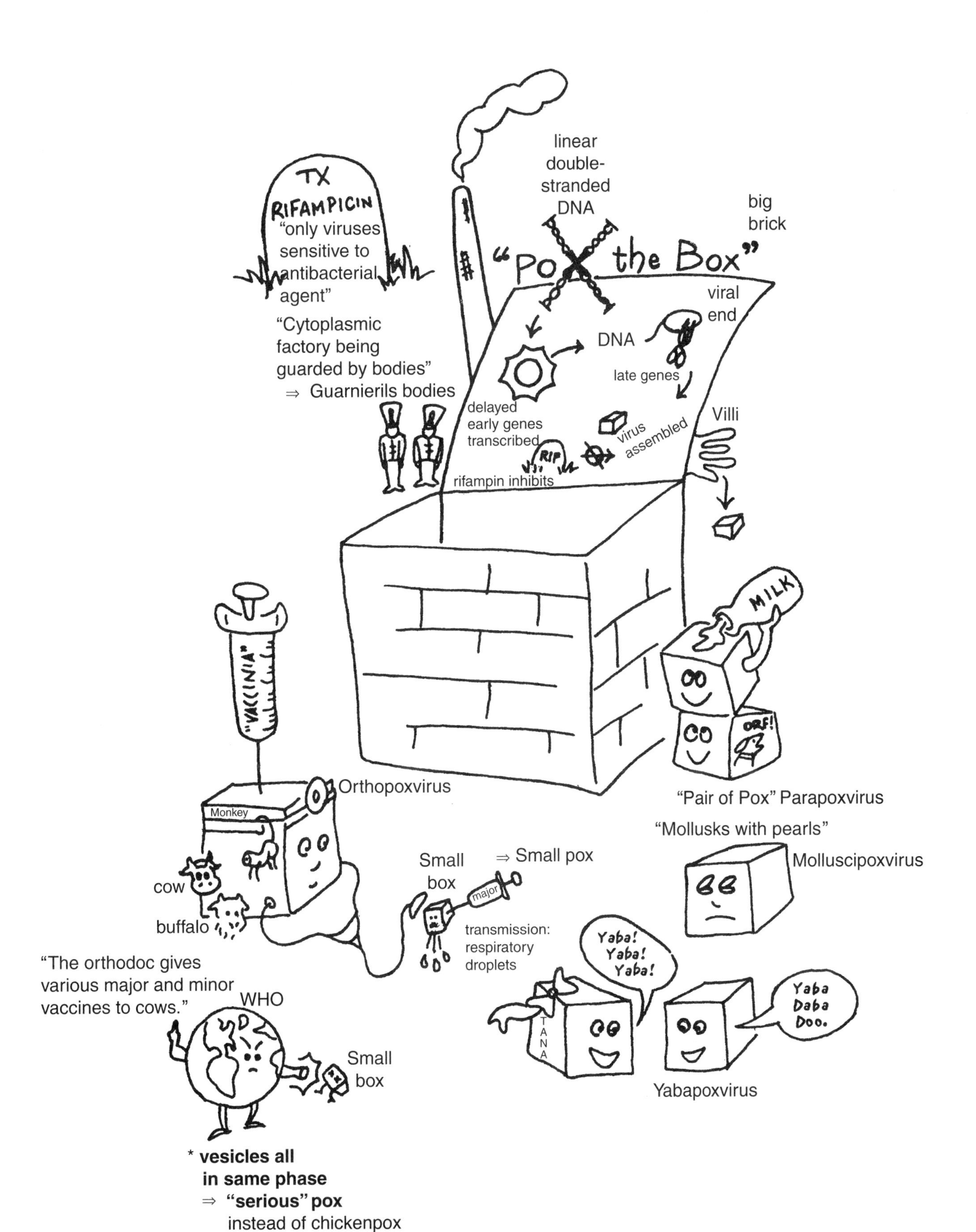
TX
RIFAMPICIN
"only viruses sensitive to antibacterial agent"
"Cytoplasmic factory being guarded by bodies"
⇒ Guarnierils bodies
linear double-stranded DNA
big brick
"Pox the Box"
viral end
DNA
late genes
delayed early genes transcribed
RIP
virus assembled
Villi
rifampin inhibits
MILK
"VACCINIA"
ORF!
Orthopoxvirus
Monkey
"Pair of Pox" Parapoxvirus
"Mollusks with pearls"
Molluscipoxvirus
Small box
⇒ Small pox
major
cow
buffalo
transmission: respiratory droplets
Yaba! Yaba! Yaba!
Yaba Daba Doo.
"The orthodoc gives various major and minor vaccines to cows."
WHO
Small box
TANA
Yabapoxvirus
* vesicles all in same phase
⇒ "serious" pox instead of chickenpox

HEPATITIS B (HBV)

Structure

- primary cause of serum hepatitis; hepatitis B surface antigen a.k.a. "Australian antigen"
- enveloped, small circular, partially dsDNA (with one complete strand and one partially complete); smallest animal DNA virus known

NOTES

- genome encodes only 4 proteins:
  S→surface envelope antigen (HBsAg) with forms S, M, and L
  C→core antigen (HBeAg) with form C called E (HBeAg)
  X→transcriptional activator
  P→polymerase with reverse transcriptase activity and DNAP function
- HBV replicates through RNA intermediate
- stable virion; resist ether, freezing, heating, and low pH
- HBsAg particles (incomplete virions lacking genome→Dane particles) are released into serum
- glycoproteins carry group-specific antigen (*a*) and one each of two pairs of type-specific determinants (*dy* or *wr*)→ epidemiologic markers (are significant because of rare strains of HBV that lack *a*)→*a* is the epitope with which protective antibody is made→therefore, HBV strain can be transmitted to HBV-immune individual

Replication

- defined tropism for liver hepatocytes→ attaches by HBsAg→transported to cell nucleus→host enzymes complete partial DNA strand→host RNAP transcribes 4 mRNAs and an RNA template→released into cytoplasm→template RNA encapsidated in HBcAg→RNA template transcribed into DNA→HBV DNAP begins synthesis of (+) sense DNA strand→ envelopment of nucleocapsid in HBsAg stops polymerase activity and 2nd DNA strand remains incomplete
- genome can integrate into host cell which is associated with **hepatocellular carcinoma**
- large quantities of HBsAg secreted→act as **antigenic decoys** which tie up antibodies produced (immune complexes)

Pathogenesis and Immunity

- disease acute, chronic, symptomatic, or asymptomatic→determined by patients' immune response; anti-HBs antibody protects from infection→but CMI causes liver damage
- virus replicates in liver; HBV can integrate into chromosome; intracellular build-up of HBsAg produces ground-glass hepatocyte appearance
- Interferon (INF) production by infected cells→immune response→strong CD8+ T-cell response leads to cell damage
- initial dose of HBV determines amount of cellular damage (parenchymal degeneration, cellular swelling, and necrosis→around central vein of lobule); regeneration follows resolution
- viral persistence results in chronic hepatitis→leads to cirrhosis or primary hepatocellular carcinoma
- additional damage produced by antibody-dependent cell-mediated cytotoxicity against cells' HBcAg
- immune complexes followed by hypersensitivity reactions→serum-sickness-like syndrome
- fulminant infection: escape immune response→overwhelms liver→permanent damage, cirrhosis, or death (administration of corticosteroids to stop CMI can lead to fulminant infection)

Epidemiology

- many infections transmitted from mother to infant resulting in life-long chronic infection
- infection virus in blood, semen, saliva, breast milk, vaginal secretions, and amnionic fluid→anyone coming into contact with these fluids can be at risk (including healthcare workers)

Clinical Syndromes

- **acute infection:** long incubation with insidious onset→prodrome due to immune complexes→preicteric phase→anicteric/icteric phase→recovery (4 weeks to 1 year)
- fulminant hepatitis: occurs in 1% of icteric patients; ascites and hemorrhage; death in 10 days; associated with infection with hepatitis D virus
- **chronic infection:** following recovery of asymptomatic or mild disease; chronic persistent hepatitis (no clinical signs except increased liver enzymes and antibodies); chronic active hepatitis continuous hepatic damage and regeneration of liver cells; some die of cirrhosis and some progress to primary hepatic carcinoma
- **primary hepatocellular carcinoma (PHC):** highest incidence with HBV or HCV, caused by HBV induction of continual cell growth and repair and HBV X gene product transactivates protein kinase C which deregulates expression of cellular oncogenes
- **combined HBV/HDV infection:** co-infection (more severe than HBV alone) or superinfection (HDV follows HBV infection)

Diagnosis

serologic testing for HBV antigens or antibody; HBsAg first marker present indicates active infection; HBeAg and HBV DNA indicate active infection, high viremia, and infectivity; anti-HBs antibody indicates immunity or recovery; anti-HBc antibody indicates present or past infection; anti-HBc-IgM indicates current infection; anti-HBe antibody indicates low infectivity

Treatment

no specific antiviral treatment; **DO NOT USE CORTICOSTEROIDS**; prevention with vaccine; control by using universal blood and body fluid precautions

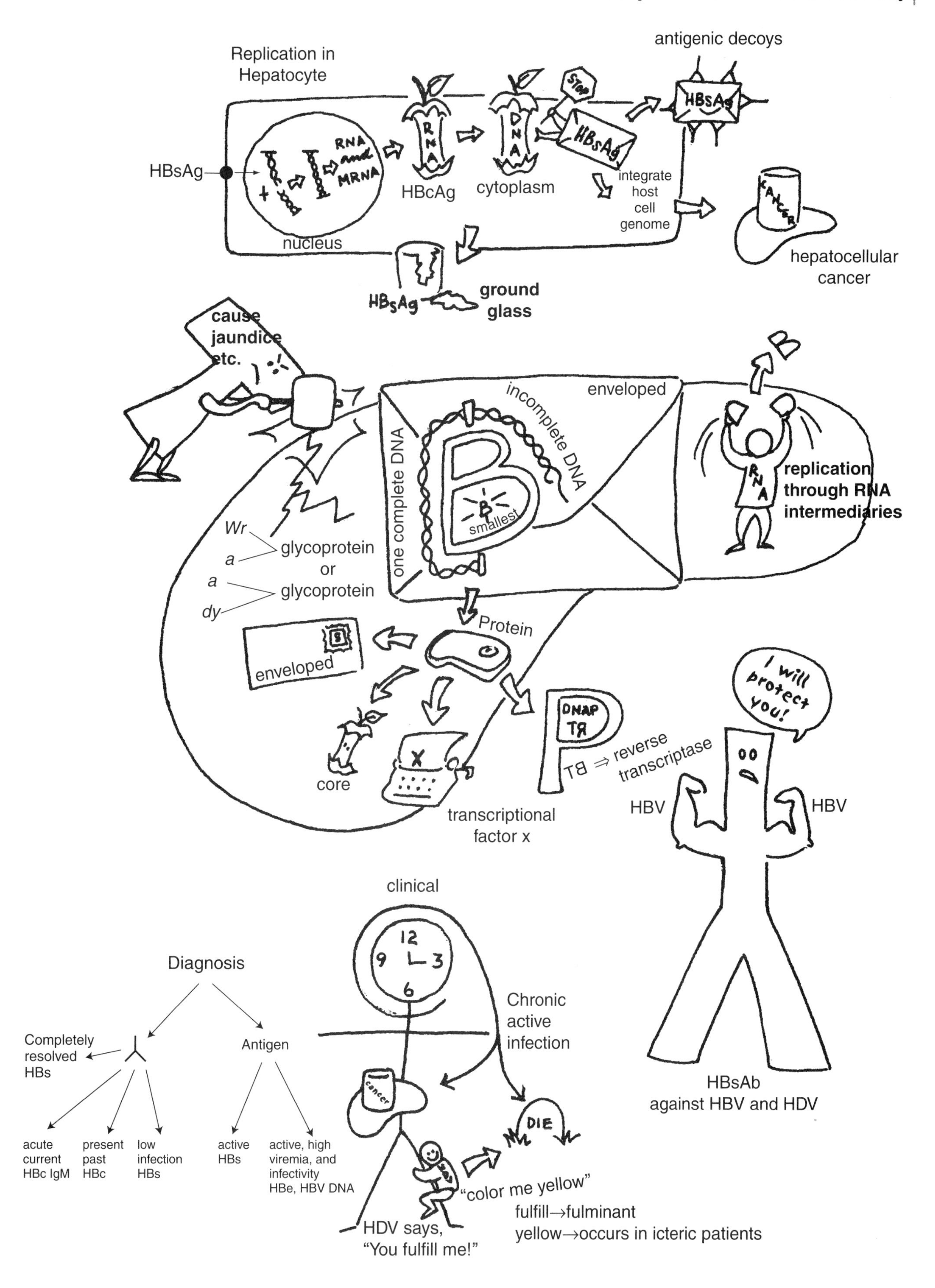
Replication in Hepatocyte
antigenic decoys
HBsAg
RNA and MRNA
HBcAg
cytoplasm
STOP
HBsAg
integrate host cell genome
nucleus
CANCER
hepatocellular cancer
HBsAg
ground glass
cause jaundice etc.
enveloped
incomplete DNA
one complete DNA
smallest
B
replication through RNA intermediaries
Wr
a
a
dy
glycoprotein
or
glycoprotein
Protein
enveloped
core
DNAP
TR
TB ⇒ reverse transcriptase
transcriptional factor x
I will protect you!
HBV
HBV
HBsAb against HBV and HDV
clinical
12
9
3
6
Chronic active infection
Diagnosis
Completely resolved HBs
Antigen
acute current HBc IgM
present past HBc
low infection HBs
active HBs
active, high viremia, and infectivity HBe, HBV DNA
cancer
DIE
"color me yellow"
fulfill→fulminant
yellow→occurs in icteric patients
HDV says, "You fulfill me!"

HEPATITIS

- 5 types: A, B, C, D, E
- all cause similar clinical picture: hepatitis, hepatocellular necrosis, jaundice, and/or release of liver enzymes don't affect other organs
- **classic viral hepatitis:** jaundice (icterus), elevated liver transaminases (AST, ALT), low fever, nausea and vomiting, fatigue, depression, and anorexia
- **anticteric infection (without jaundice):** anorexia, malaise, fever, abnormal AST and ALT
- **asymptomatic infections**

HEPATITIS A (HAV)

Structure

HAV belongs to **Picornaviridae;** icosahedral, nonenveloped, linear ss (+)RNA genome; only one serotype

Pathogenesis

- ingested→replicates in intestinal epithelial cells→spreads via the bloodstream or lymph to liver→establishes a persistent noncytolytic infection of the parenchymal cells→virus shed in feces before symptoms→CTLs cause liver damage→ does not establish a chronic infection or cholestasis
- immunity after recovery is lifelong

Epidemiology

- one of most stable viruses known to infect humans; resistant to acid pH of 1, detergents, organic solvents, and high temperatures; stable in dried feces for 30 days
- transmitted by fecal-oral route; endemic where sanitation is poor
- outbreaks usually have common source; food

NOTES

Clinical Syndromes

- hepatitis onset is abrupt
- first 2 weeks: fatigue, nausea and vomiting, anorexia, upper right quadrant pain, myalgia
- during 3rd week jaundice and itching appear as other symptoms decline

Diagnosis

elevated liver enzymes; HAV specific IgM (onset and first 3–6 months); replaced by specific IgG

Treatment

symptomatic; prophylaxis with Ig; killed-virus vaccine; prevention

HEPATITIS C (HCV)

General

- belongs to family **Flaviviridae**
- icosahedral, enveloped with ss(+)RNA nonsegmented genome
- establishes noncytolytic, persistent infection that results in chronic disease
- hypervariable regions of glycoproteins E1 and E2 account for development of different serotypes of virus

Epidemiology

- common in IV drug users; parenteral and sexual transmission

Clinical Syndrome

- 75% of cases are subclinical; similar to HBV symptoms except less severe; little or no jaundice; infection marked by widely fluctuating serum ALT levels
- can develop chronic persistent hepatitis with continuous viremia for over 10 years; chronic infection may progress to cirrhosis or cancer
- antibody developed in course of infection is not protective

Diagnosis

EIA tests; detection of HCV RNA in blood

Treatment

recombinant INF-α

HEPATITIS D (HDV)

- viral parasite
- only member of **Deltavirus** genus
- a.k.a. Delta agent
- HBsAg required for packaging virus

Structure

- smallest animal RNA known; encodes one protein; RNA genome surrounded by delta antigen covered with HBsAg
- circularized and rod-shaped ss(–)RNA

Replication

- host cell RNAP II copies RNA→RNA genome forms ribosyme→cleaves RNA circle and forms mRNA→mRNA translated to small delta antigen→cellular enzyme mutates delta gene to produce large delta antigen

Pathogenesis

- spread same as HBV; HBV infection must already be present or acquired at the same time for disease to occur (co-infection or **superinfection**); HDV replication→liver damage; antibodies occur but not protective; protective antibodies are anti-HBs antibodies

Epidemiology

- mirrors HBV but less common

Clinical Syndromes

- increases HBV infection severity
- fulminant hepatitis; chronic infection occurs in individuals with chronic HBV infection

Diagnosis

antibodies to delta antigen

Treatment

none

HEPATITIS E (HEV)

Structure

- belongs to family **Caliciviridae**
- spherical, nonenveloped, and genome is nonsegmented ss(+)RNA
- less environmentally stable

Pathogenesis

- similar symptoms as HAV except cholestasis included→intracanalicular stasis of bile associated with rosette formation of hepatocytes and pseudoglandular structures resembling embryonal bile ducts

Epidemiology

- transmission via fecal-oral route through contaminated water
- increased mortality in pregnant women especially if contracted during 3rd trimester

Clinical Syndromes

- children asymptomatic and adults become icteric; no chronic hepatitis; no carrier state; no association with cirrhosis or cancer

Diagnosis

exclusion of HAV, HBV, HCV

Treatment

none

- **HFV similar to HEV**
- **new HGV; flavivirus found in patients with nonA, nonB, and nonC hepatitis**

Hepatitis A, C, D, and E (Liver)

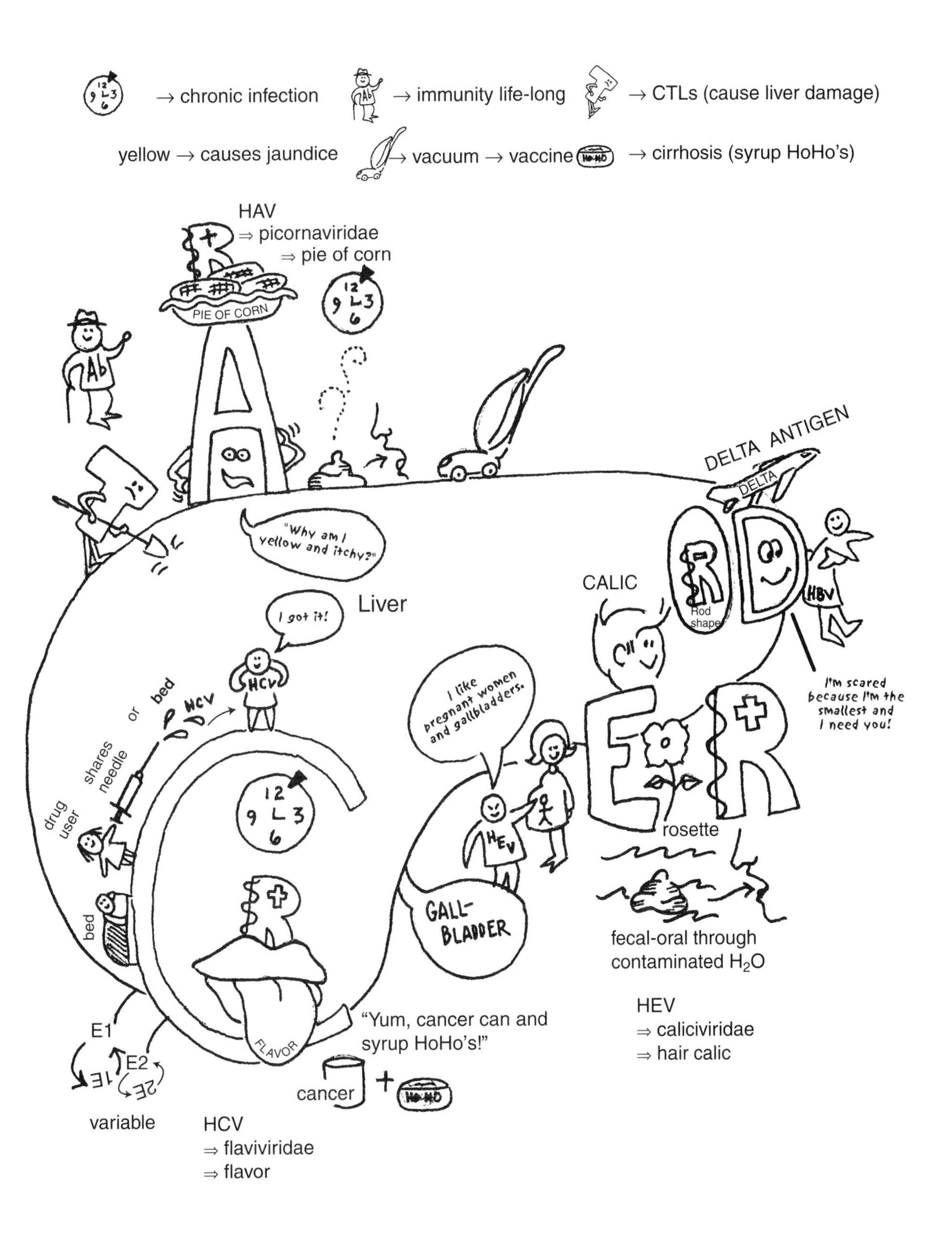

PICORNAVIRIDAE

⇒ "Pie of Corn"

Structure

- small, icosahedral, nonenveloped linear ss(+)RNA, nonsegmented; 3′ polyA tail and 5′ VPg protein; genome infectious; no transcriptase in nucleocapsid
- entire genome translated into a complex polyprotein→cleave into smaller proteins; complex capsid proteins (VP1–4)
- 3 of 5 genera pathogenic: enterovirus, rhinovirus, hepatovirus (HAV)

Replication

- attachment via VP1 (CSR lies within protective canyon→antibodies cannot reach); ICAM-1 CSR for rhinovirus; IgG for poliovirus; VLA-2 for echovirus
- enters via endocytosis or channel→upon entry translation begins immediately→viral RNAP generates a (–) strand template from which (+) sense genomes/mRNAs are synthesized→more negative templates→released by cell lysis

NOTES

ENTEROVIRUS

(includes poliovirus, coxsackievirus, echovirus, enterovirus)

Pathogenesis

- enters oropharynx and replicates→pass through stomach to intestine and replicate again→may spread to lymph
- primary viremia disseminates to target tissues recognized by specific adhesions; replication in target tissue causes local damage→symptoms are related to infected tissue and secondary viremia
- antibody is immune response and is protective; CMI not involved in protection but pathogenesis (especially coxsackievirus B myocarditis)

Epidemiology

- affect humans only; increased incidence of polio paralytic disease with advancing age
- transmitted by fecal-oral route; virus shed for months from intestine; secondary transmission by contact with feces or contact with flies; respiratory droplets also transmit
- stable in environment; peak incidence in summer to fall

Clinical Diseases

CNS DISEASES

- **aseptic meningitis:** uneventful unless accompanied by encephalitis or in infants
- **paralysis:** poliomyelitis and enterovirus 70 and 71; follows or occurs with aseptic meningitis
- **poliomyelitis:** poliovirus 1–3; infection limited to oropharynx and intestine is asymptomatic; remainder have biphasic disease→first phase is mild illness then second phase begins with aseptic meningitis and stops or spreads to spinal or bulbar
- paralytic poliomyelitis: spinal poliomyelitis affects muscles innervated by spinal cord; bulbar polio affects cranial nerves and is associated with respiratory paralysis
- **postpolio syndrome:** occurs 30–40 years later to original victims→deterioration of originally affected muscles caused by loss of originally infected neurons
- **chronic meningoencephalitis with juvenile dermatomyositis:** fatal disease in immunodeficient children
- **eye infections:** enterovirus 70, coxsackievirus A24: acute hemorrhagic conjunctivitis
- **myocarditis:** coxsackievirus B
- **pleurodynia (Bornholm disease, epidemic myalgia, devil's grip):** coxsackie B1-6, coxsackie A, echovirus: abrupt onset of chest pain in lower ribs or sternum with stabbing pain and cough, may radiate
- **respiratory tract infection:** coxsackie A21, A24, B1-6, echovirus 11: febrile colds with sore throat; seen in summer
- **skin and mucosal infection: hand-foot-and-mouth disease:** coxsackie A9, A16, enterovirus 71; seen in children, vesicular eruption in mouth, periungual area of hands and heel margins; shallow white lesion with red areolae
- **herpangina:** coxsackie A: severe febrile pharyngitis with grayish white vesicles; throat very red
- **maculopapular exanthems-enterovirus:** transient and no complications; mimics rubella, roseola, or rubeola
- **other enteroviral infection:→juvenile-onset insulin-dependent diabetes; hemolytic-uremic syndrome; neonatal disease** (often fatal with encephalomyocarditis syndrome and hemorrhagic hepatitis syndrome)

Diagnosis

cell culture; meningitis: examine CSF to rule out bacteria; PCR for aseptic meningitis and encephalitis from CSF; viral meningitis high lymphocytes and bacterial meningitis high polymorphonuclear leukocytes (PMNs)

Treatment

supportive only; prevention with polio vaccine (live/Sabin and killed/Salk trivalent); gut immunity important

RHINOVIRUS

- labile at pH 3 and prefer to replicate at 33–35°C; inactivated at 37°C→restricts virus to upper airways

Pathogenesis and Immunity

- use ICAM-1 as CSR; symptoms relate to quantity of virus shed;
- infected cells secrete bradykinin and histamine→causes runny nose and upregulates ICAM-1→increasing viral invasion; resolves with specific IgA; however, protection is only for a short time

Epidemiology

- account for 50% of common colds; early fall and late spring
- transmission: human to human, fomites, respiratory droplet→infection only requires one particle

Clinical Syndrome

- common cold: if fever develops indicates secondary infection; may cause tracheobronchitis or pneumonia

Diagnosis

rarely pursued

Treatment

no antiviral treatment; avoid antipyretic agents because enhances shedding of virus; encourage prevention

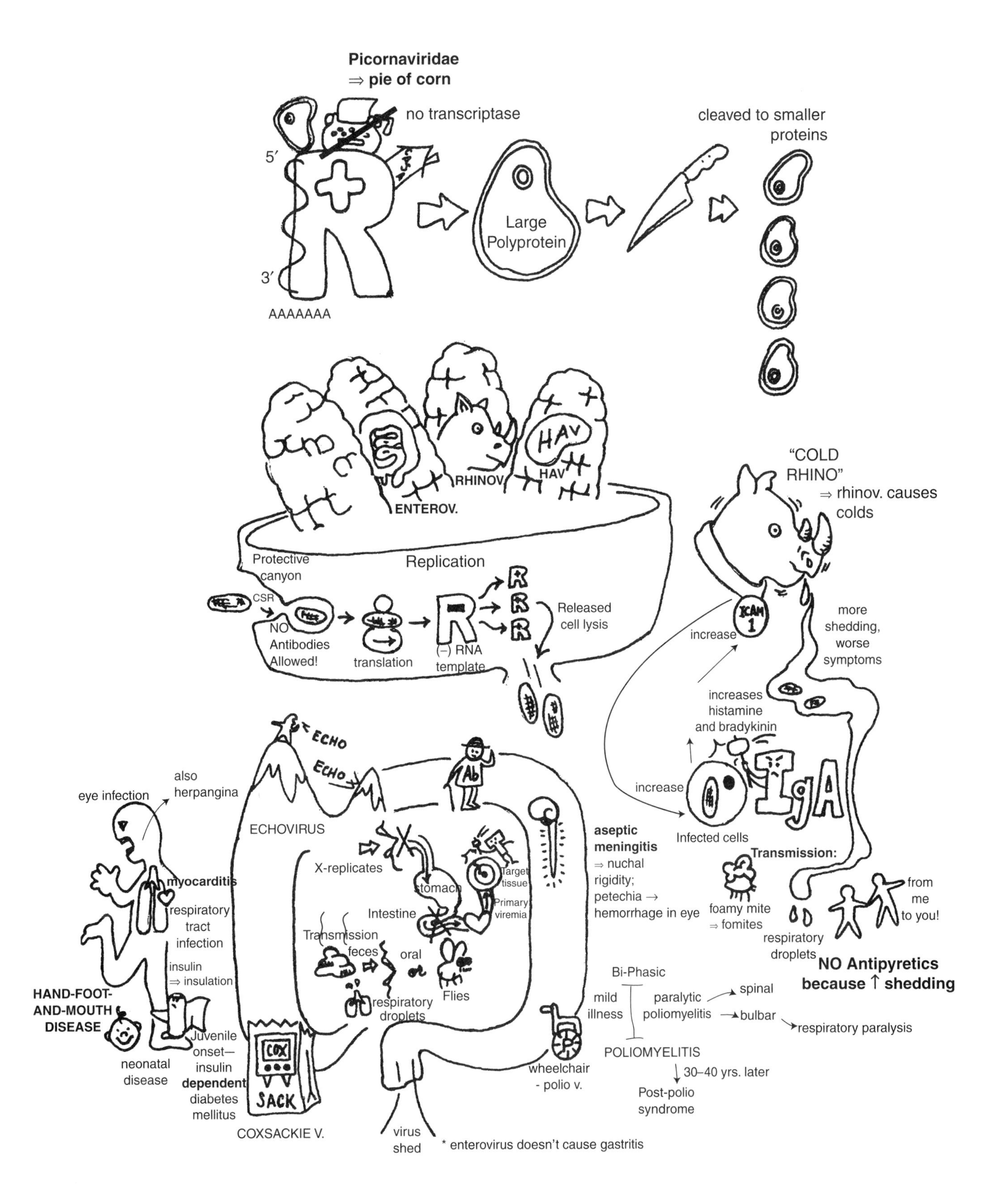
Picornaviridae
⇒ pie of corn
no transcriptase
5′
3′
AAAAAAA
Large
Polyprotein
cleaved to smaller
proteins
HAV
RHINOV
HAV
ENTEROV.
"COLD
RHINO"
⇒ rhinov. causes
colds
Protective
canyon
Replication
CSR
NO
Antibodies
Allowed!
translation
(–) RNA
template
Released
cell lysis
increase
more
shedding,
worse
symptoms
increases
histamine
and bradykinin
increase
Infected cells
Transmission:
foamy mite
⇒ fomites
respiratory
droplets
from
me
to you!
NO Antipyretics
because ↑ shedding
ECHO
ECHO
ECHOVIRUS
eye infection
also
herpangina
myocarditis
respiratory
tract
infection
insulin
⇒ insulation
HAND-FOOT-
AND-MOUTH
DISEASE
neonatal
disease
Juvenile
onset—
insulin
dependent
diabetes
mellitus
COX
SACK
COXSACKIE V.
X-replicates
Stomach
Target
tissue
Primary
viremia
Intestine
Transmission
feces
oral
or
Flies
respiratory
droplets
aseptic
meningitis
⇒ nuchal
rigidity;
petechia →
hemorrhage in eye
Bi-Phasic
mild
illness
paralytic
poliomyelitis
spinal
bulbar
respiratory paralysis
POLIOMYELITIS
30–40 yrs. later
Post-polio
syndrome
wheelchair
- polio v.
virus
shed
* enterovirus doesn't cause gastritis

NOTES

CALICIVIRIDAE

⇒ hair calic

- includes 2 human pathogens: Norwalk viruses and HEV (**Nor**th Pole **Walk** and **HEaVy** Bag)
- small, nonenveloped, icosahedral with cup-shaped indentations
- Norwalk are more rounded than others and more resistant to chlorine, heat, and stomach acid

Pathogenesis

- attach to intestinal brush border and are internalized→inhibits water and nutrient absorption→tips of jejunal villi slough off (look blunted)→lamina propria infiltrated with mononuclear cells and PMNs→ delayed gastric emptying and transient malabsorption
- some persons naturally resistant; those who develop antibodies are only protected for a few months

Epidemiology

- transmission is fecal–oral; outbreaks have common source; patients shed virus within 2 days of infection

Clinical Disease

- **stomach "flu" or winter vomiting disease**

Diagnosis

clinically made

Treatment

symptomatic

Prevention

adequate chlorination of potable water and good hygiene

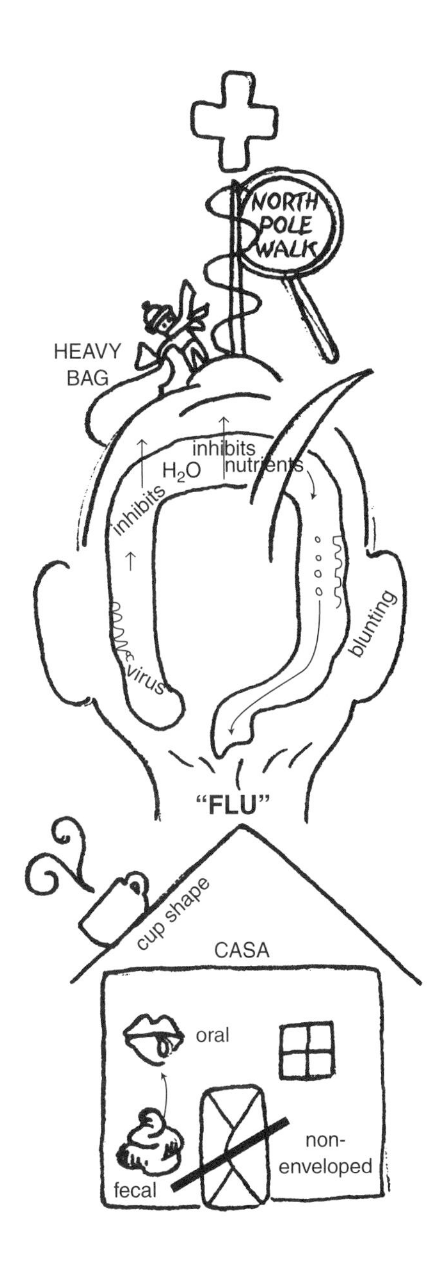
NORTH
POLE
WALK
HEAVY
BAG
inhibits
H_2O
inhibits
nutrients
virus
blunting
"FLU"
cup shape
CASA
oral
non-
enveloped
fecal

NOTES

ASTROVIRIDAE

- icosahedral, nonenveloped; appearance of 5- or 6-pointed star in EM; genome nonsegmented linear ss(+)RNA and no transcriptase—typewriter

Epidemiology

- spread by fecal–oral route (food, water, or person to person); winter

Clinical Disease

- adults and older children→no symptoms
- young children and immunocompromised→ mild gastroenteritis with watery diarrhea

Diagnosis

resolves before testing needed; EIA for viral antigen or EM

Treatment

symptomatic; prevention good hygiene

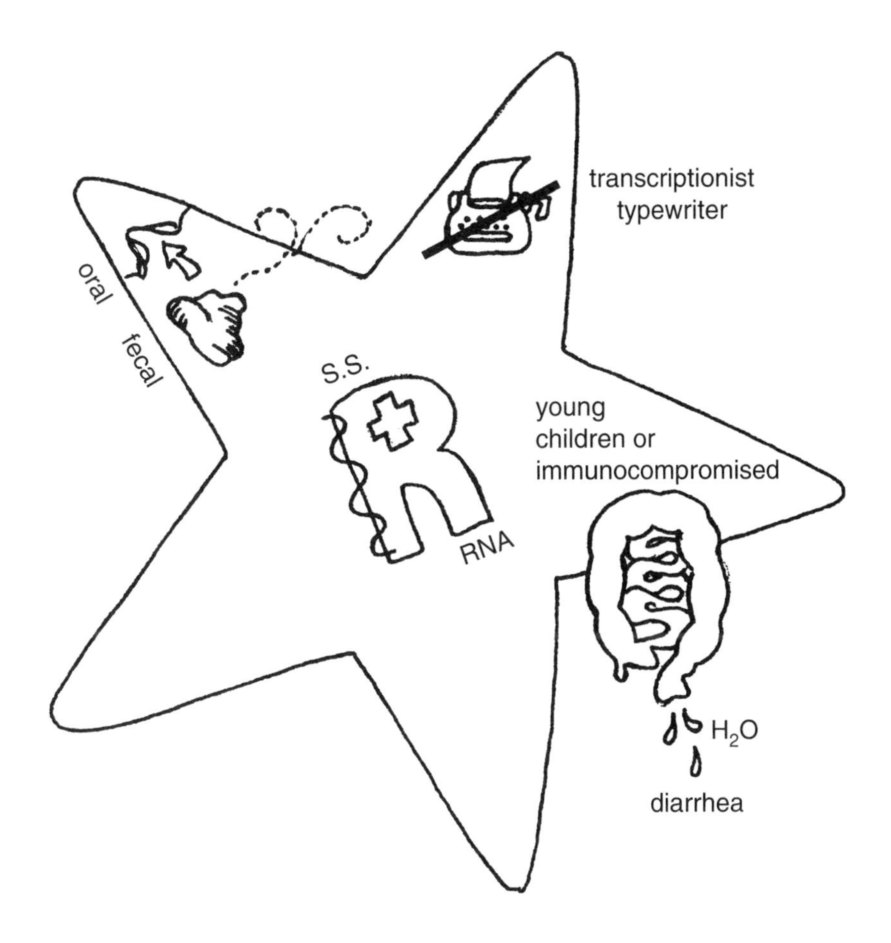
transcriptionist
typewriter
oral
fecal
S.S.
RNA
young
children or
immunocompromised
H2O
diarrhea

NOTES

CORONAVIRIDAE

⇒ crown

- primarily pathogens of mammals and birds; coronavirus and torovirus mild infection in humans; corona species can cause common cold
- largest of spherical RNAs, enveloped, helical nucleocapsid with linear ss(+)RNA, nonsegmented; no transcriptase in nucleocapsid
- club-shaped **peplomers** of glycoprotein giving the appearance of the solar corona
- nucleocapsid N-protein attached to envelope by transmembrane M protein; **viral S (spike)** protein acts as an adhesin that causes viral-cell membrane fusion (also agglutinates RBCs)

Pathogenesis

- corono. replicate in nasal epithelial cells; do not spread to bloodstream because of temperature; mechanism of pathogenesis unknown

Epidemiology

- spread by aerosols and respiratory droplets

Clinical Disease

- **common colds:** exacerbation of preexisting lung conditions
- immunity strain specific and short-lived
- found in stools of patients with **mild diarrhea or gastroenteritis** and infants with neonatal necrotizing enterocolitis

Treatment

- none

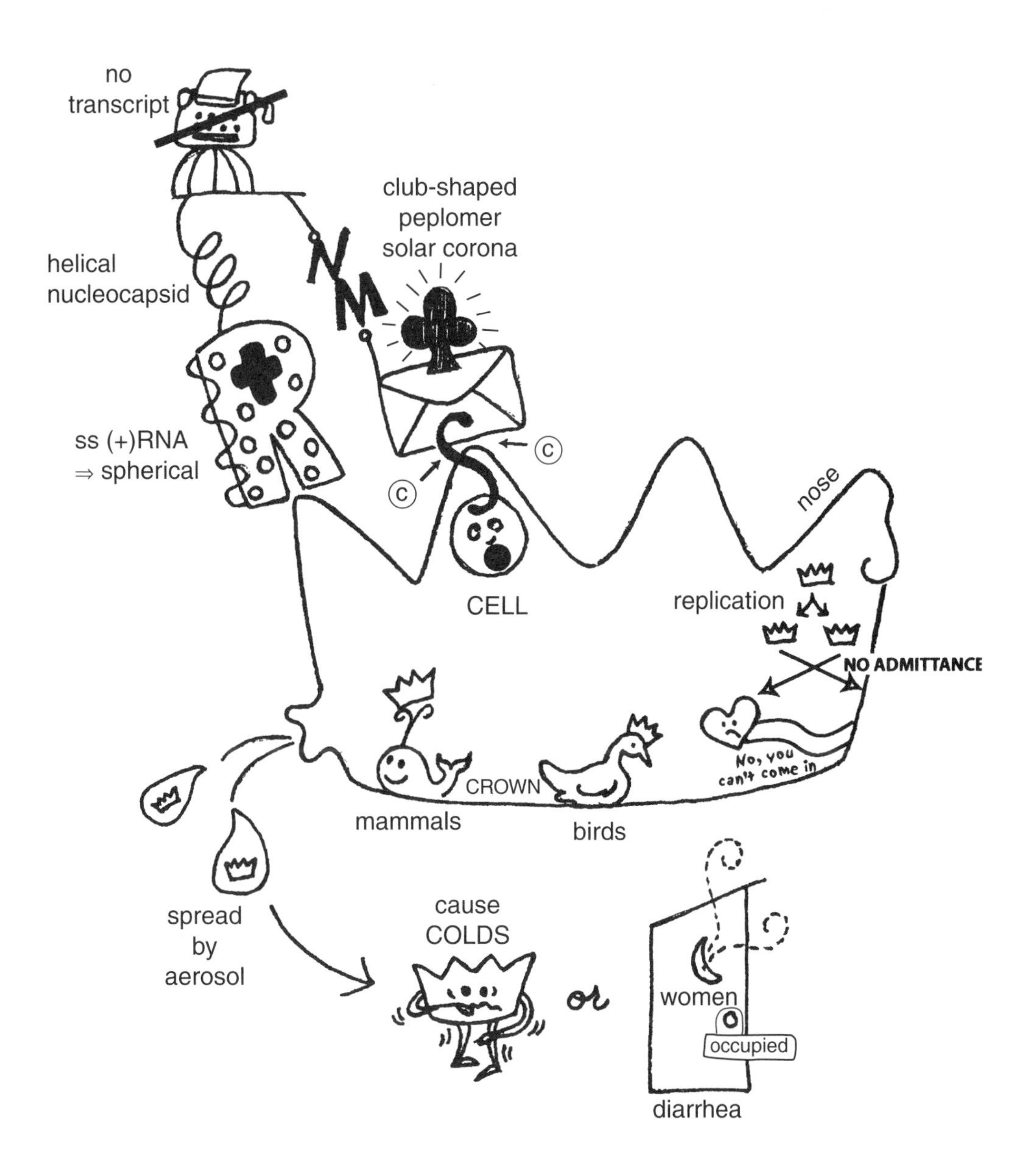
no
transcript
helical
nucleocapsid
club-shaped
peplomer
solar corona
ss (+)RNA
⇒ spherical
©
©
nose
CELL
replication
NO ADMITTANCE
No, you
can't come in
CROWN
mammals
birds
spread
by
aerosol
cause
COLDS
or
women
occupied
diarrhea

NOTES

TOGAVIRIDAE

⇒ toga

- two genera infect humans: alphavirus and rubivirus (rubella)
- enveloped, icosahedral, linear ss(+)RNA genome and nonsegmented; no transcriptase

Replication

- translation of first 2/3→polyprotein →cleaved into 4 proteins→(–)RNA template transcribed→two (+)RNA then transcribed from template→one full-length genomic RNA and one smaller RNA translated into second polyprotein→ cleaved into core protein (C) and 3 glycoproteins

ALPHAVIRUS

Pathogenesis and Immunity

- cycle (Group A arbovirus) infection includes vertebrate host (lytic infection) and invertebrate vector (persistent infection)
- mosquito bite→replication in endothelium of capillaries, macrophages, monocytes, and reticuloendothelial cells→dissemination via bloodstream to target
- initial viremia associated with flu symptoms; usually resolves because of specific IgM then IgG; symptoms occur if reaches target tissue: brain, joints, skin, or muscle

Epidemiology

- humans dead-end host
- **species of α-virus confined to specific geographical location because of the need of specific hosts and vectors for the virus to spread**
- encephalitis in Americas—spread by *Culex* or *Aedes* mosquitoes

Clinical Syndromes

- **encephalitis:** fever→nuchal rigidity→confusion and coma; eastern equine encephalitis most severe; also western and Venezuela type
- **fever with arthritis, myalgia, and rash:** high fever→severe polyarthritis affecting small joints (fingers)→rash

Diagnosis

cultured during viremia; serologic tests for specific IgM and increased IgG

Treatment

only supportive; prevention with immunization of horses; and elimination of vector

RUBIVIRUS

*only one not arthropod-borne

- causes rubella, German measles
- infection during pregnancy life-threatening for fetus

Pathogenesis and Immunity

- infection begins in upper respiratory tract→lymph nodes→viremia→ dissemination
- congenital infection: replicates in placenta and spreads to fetus→slowing down mitosis of fetal cells causing teratogenic effects (especially during 1st trimester)
- antibody appearance coincides with rash and arthralgia; life-long protective antibody occurs with one serotype (also protects against congenital infection)
- establishes persistent infection in infants who shed for up to one year; if infection during immune system development, can cause tolerance to virus and infection won't be resolved

Epidemiology

- shed in respiratory droplets; not very contagious

Clinical Diseases

- **acquired rubella:** prodrome→ lymphadenopathy→maculopapular rash that begins on face and moves down→ rash fades as it moves down and "**runs out at the feet**"
- **acute rubella encephalitis**
- **self-limiting arthritis in adult women**
- **congenital rubella:** most serious outcome; infected in utero causes severe defects; causes increase in fetal death

Diagnosis

detection of antibodies; test: women considering pregnancy and not sure of immune status, pregnant woman who develop rash, and infants with congenital rubella syndrome

Treatment and Prevention

immunization

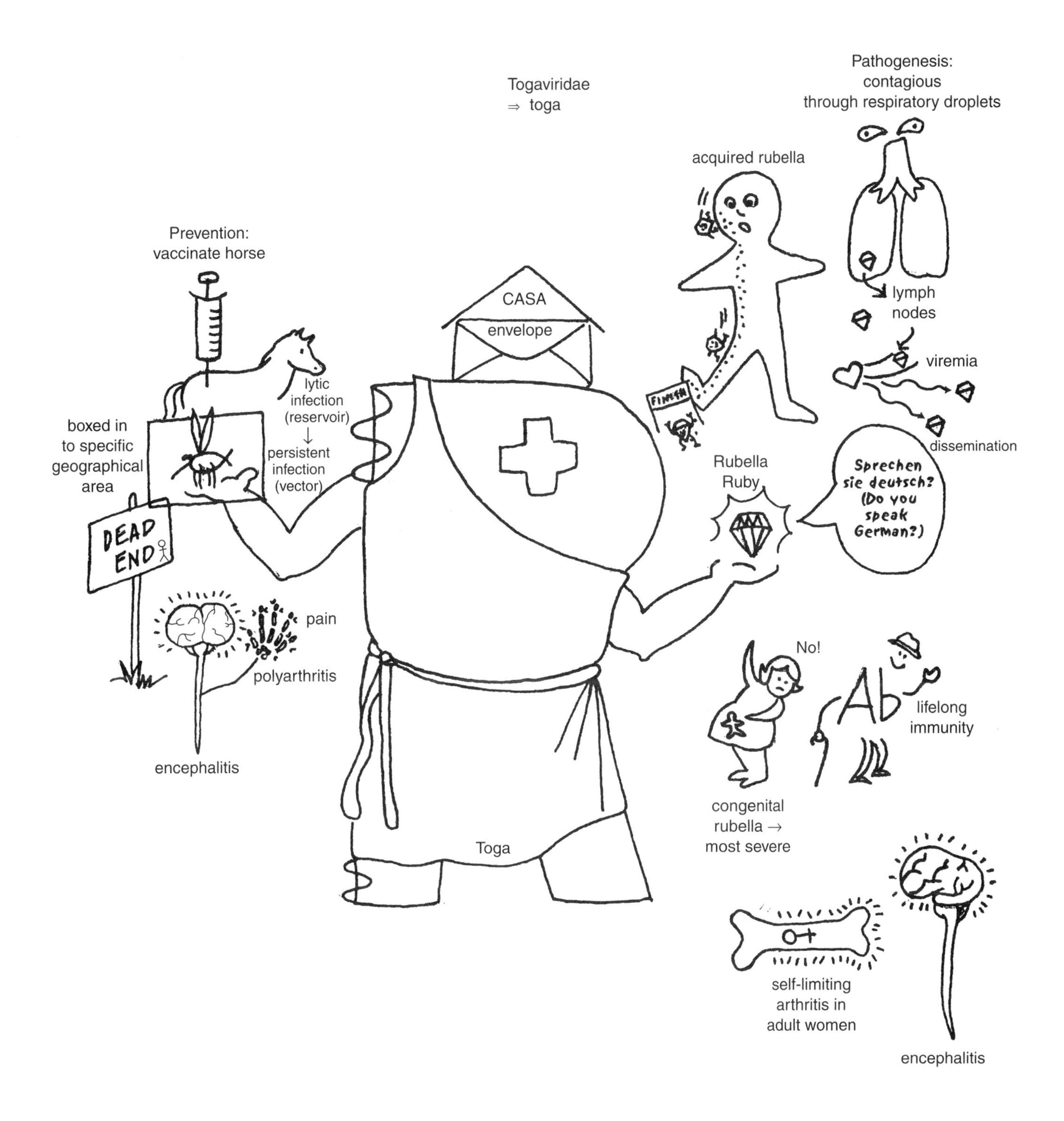
Togaviridae
⇒ toga
Pathogenesis:
contagious
through respiratory droplets
acquired rubella
lymph
nodes
viremia
dissemination
Prevention:
vaccinate horse
CASA
envelope
lytic
infection
(reservoir)
↓
persistent
infection
(vector)
boxed in
to specific
geographical
area
DEAD
END
FINISH
Rubella
Ruby
Sprechen
sie deutsch?
(Do you
speak
German?)
pain
polyarthritis
encephalitis
No!
Ab
lifelong
immunity
congenital
rubella →
most severe
Toga
self-limiting
arthritis in
adult women
encephalitis

NOTES

FLAVIVIRIDAE

- 3 genera: flavivirus, pestivirus, and HCV; only **flavivirus** and **HCV** human pathogen; flavivirus arthropod borne (group B arboviruses)
- cause fevers with arthritis, myalgia and rash, hemorrhagic fevers, or encephalitis
- flavivirus are enveloped, icosahedral, ss(+)RNA genome that is nonsegmented and infectious by itself
- single capsid protein and one envelope glycoprotein peplomer→adhesin
- entry by interaction of peplomer with CSR or via antibody-mediated uptake when virus is coated with non-neutralizing antibody; **promotes viral uptake by the cellular Fc receptors and enhances viral infectivity**
- **flavivirus replicate within perinuclear foci and are assembled in the cisternae of the ER→escape by cell lysis**

Pathogenesis and Immunity

- **yellow fever virus** (hemorrhagic fever virus): replicates in Kupffer cells in liver; massive necrosis of hepatocytes→icterus and decrease in prothrombin production; patient jaundiced, GI hemorrhage, hypotensive shock, petechiae, etc.
- **dengue virus** (fever, arthritis, myalgia, rash): hemorrhagic fever if patient previously infected with dengue type 1, 3, or 4 then becomes infected with type 2; Fc-mediated viral uptake enhances infection
- **Japanese encephalitis virus:** cerebral edema, congestion, hemorrhage, and extensive neuronal necrosis

Epidemiology

- flavivirus maintained in vertebrate host reservoirs and spread by arthropod vectors; mosquito→yellow fever, Japanese encephalitis, St. Louis encephalitis and dengue; birds are reservoirs for flavivirus except Japanese encephalitis (pigs) and dengue and yellow fever (monkeys); viruses maintain jungle cycle (only animals infected) and urban cycle (only humans infected)

Clinical Syndromes

- **encephalitis:** most important are Japanese and St. Louis types
- **fever with arthritis, myalgia, and rash:** caused by dengue and West Nile fever virus; **a.k.a. break bone fever due to intense pain of bones**; fever then rash; itching on palms of hands and soles of feet; loss of taste; if hemorrhage does not occur patient survives
- **hemorrhagic fever:** caused by yellow fever virus, dengue viruses (if patient's first infection is followed by infection with type 2); yellow fever—subclinical to fatal within 5 days; abrupt onset of fever; jaundice on 3rd day; degeneration of liver, kidney, and heart, bleeding from gums, nose, and GI (black vomit)
- **dengue hemorrhagic fever (DHF):** fever followed by cyanosis, dyspnea, ecchymoses, epistaxis, etc.

Diagnosis

arboviruses should be isolated to determine type; IgG titers and IgM; EIA

Treatment

none other than supportive
Prevention: eradication of vectors; vaccine for yellow fever and Japanese encephalitis; none for dengue

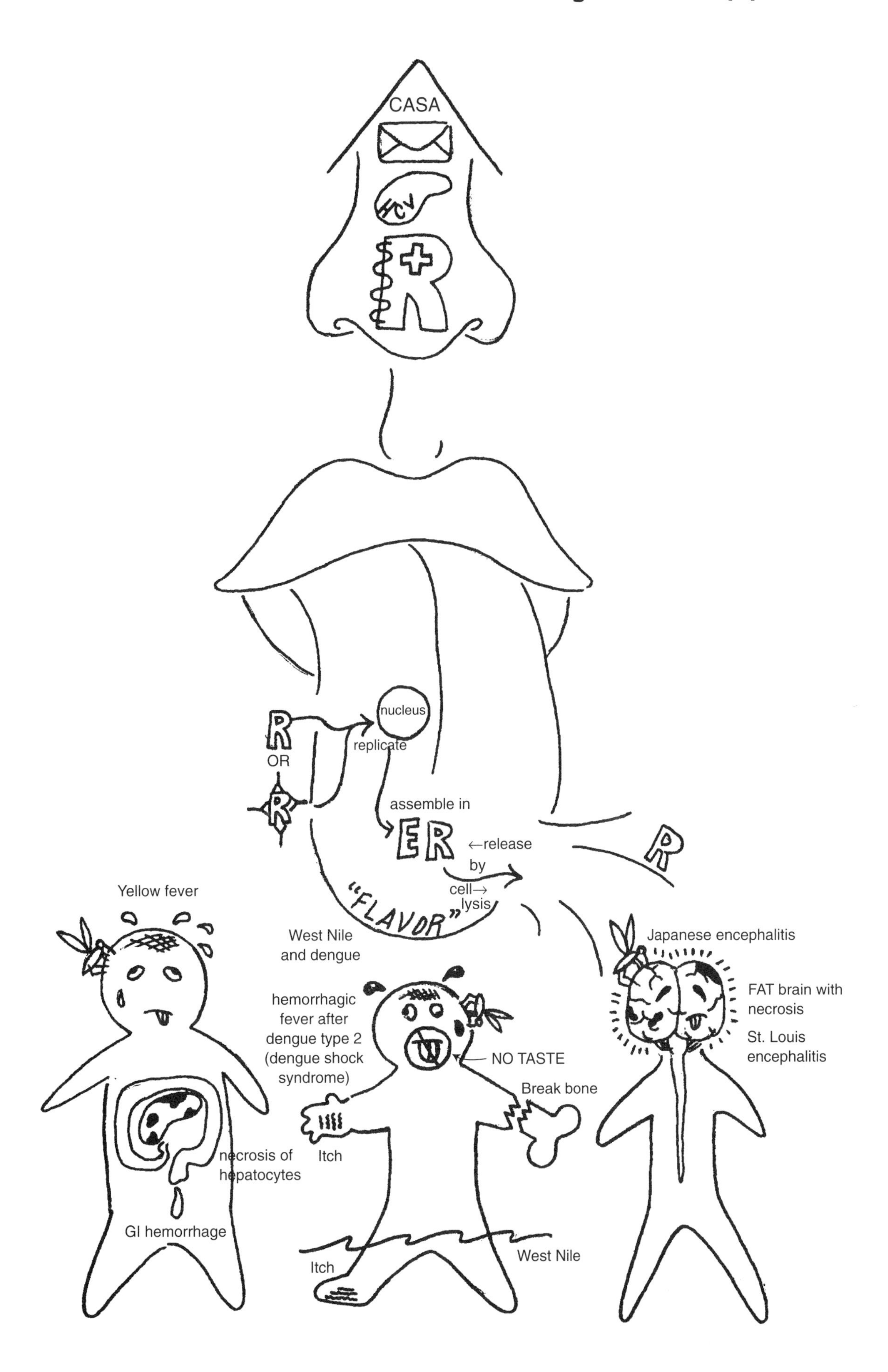
CASA
HCV
nucleus
replicate
OR
assemble in
ER
←release
by
cell→
lysis
"FLAVOR"
Yellow fever
necrosis of
hepatocytes
GI hemorrhage
West Nile
and dengue
hemorrhagic
fever after
dengue type 2
(dengue shock
syndrome)
NO TASTE
Break bone
Itch
Itch
West Nile
Japanese encephalitis
FAT brain with
necrosis
St. Louis
encephalitis

RNA Viruses: Segmented Single-Stranded (–) RNA

NOTES

Orthomyxoviridae, Bunyaviridae, Arenaviridae

- segmented have 2–10 separate strands of RNA, each encoding a single viral protein; genome not infectious; virion must include viral RNA-dependent RNAP
- **genetic shift:** closely related viruses infect cell at same time→genomes mix together resulting in hybrid→functional new virus may appear

Replication

- ribonucleoprotein core to nucleus→(–) RNAs are transcribed to construct mRNAs and complete (+)copies of genome→ RNAP steals caps and nucleotides from cellular mRNAs to use as primers to initiate viral mRNA synthesis→translation of these mRNAs→viral proteins; genomic replication→after NP attaches binds to (–) strands; the RNAP copies (–) strand to (+) strands and then copies another (–) strand
- release occurs through budding
- **defective interfering particles (DIPs):** many defective virions are released that are incomplete yet can bind to CSRs→interfering with entry and replication of complete infectious virions

ORTHOMYXOVIRIDAE

- influenzavirus A, B, C; tick-borne viruses Dhori and Thogoto
- enveloped; contain 6–8 helical nucleocapsids; nucleoprotein (NP) and RNAP; **M1→maintains shape; M2→ion channel in envelope; envelope contains H hemagglutinin and N neuraminidase**

Pathogenesis

- attach via H protein to sialic acid receptors on host cell→endocytosis→endosome pH falls to 5.5→H changes form and causes fusion of the viral envelope with endosomal membrane→**protons pass through M2**→causes nucleocapsids to be released into cytosol→transported to nucleus where transcription and replication occur
- infect ciliary columnar epithelial cells of airway→tracheobronchitis and bronchospasms
- **viral neuraminidase N thins mucus and slows ciliary action→viruses travel to lungs in thinned secretions; desquamation of bronchial or alveolar epithelial cells down to BM; hyaline membranes can occur in lung→alveolar emphysema and necrosis**
- **infection initiates antiviral state;** antibody develops against H→neutralizes virus→prevents infection; resolution occurs with INF and CMI (delayed because virus depresses T-cell function)
- influenza A virus can undergo **antigenic shift** (mixing of 2 virus types leads to production of new H); types A and B→ **antigenic drift** (point mutation of H receptor therefore neutralizing antibodies are no longer effective)

Epidemiology

- pandemics frequently begin in SE Asia when recombinant virus arises from infected ducks or swine; the more the antigens change the more cases will occur in outbreak
- spread by airborne droplets; survive 24 hrs on fomites; contagion precedes symptoms

Clinical Syndromes

- acute influenza in adult
- acute influenza in children: higher fever and croup frequently occur
- influenza most severe in elderly: persistent cough, pneumonia
- complications: primary viral pneumonia, secondary bacterial pneumonia, Reye's syndrome, Guillain-Barré syndrome

Diagnosis

clinical

Treatment

symptomatic treatment: rest, fluids, and antipyretic agents (do not use aspirin→Reye's syndrome); **amantadine** and **rimantadine** decrease severity if given first 48 hrs; amantadine also prophylactic

- **killed virus trivalent vaccines**

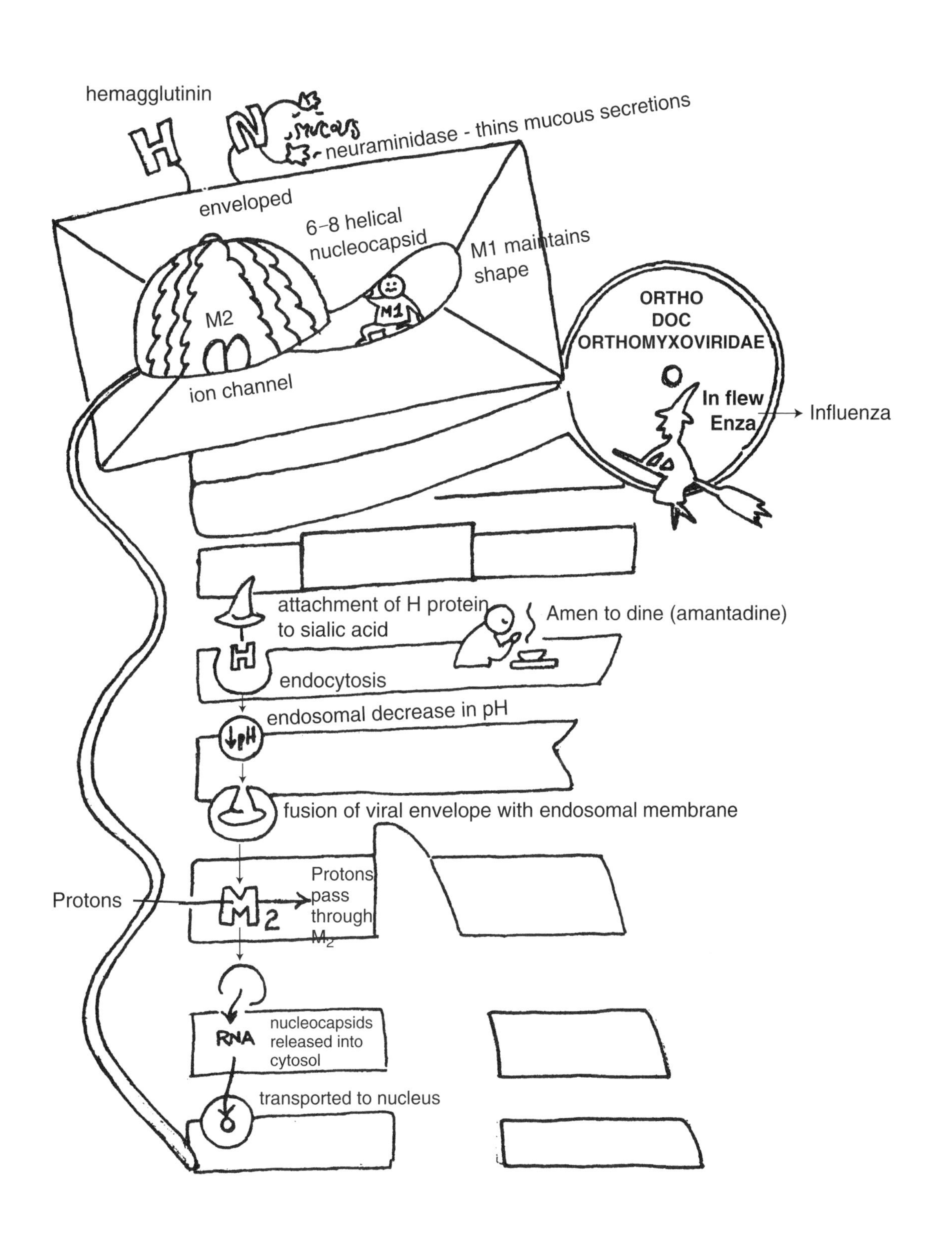
hemagglutinin
H
N
mucus
neuraminidase - thins mucous secretions
enveloped
6–8 helical nucleocapsid
M1 maintains shape
M1
M2
ion channel
ORTHO
DOC
ORTHOMYXOVIRIDAE
In flew
Enza
Influenza
attachment of H protein to sialic acid
Amen to dine (amantadine)
H
endocytosis
endosomal decrease in pH
↓pH
fusion of viral envelope with endosomal membrane
Protons
M2
Protons pass through M2
RNA
nucleocapsids released into cytosol
transported to nucleus

RNA Viruses: Nonsegmented Single-Stranded (–) RNA

- nonsegmented, single-stranded (–)RNA, enveloped, helical
- host cell cannot transcribe (–)RNA; naked genome is not infective; must include viral RNA-dependent RNAP in capsid

PARAMYXOVIRIDAE

⇒ pair of rams

(paramyxovirus, rubulavirus, and morbillivirus)

- nucleocapsid constructed of nucleoprotein (N or NP); contains transcriptases L and P; genome surrounded by matrix protein M; envelope glycoproteins→F (fusion protein) and HN (attachment protein)

Replication

- takes place in cytoplasm; released by budding; as F inserts into cell membrane→ infected cells merge with adjacent cells to form syncytia (giant cells)
- HN is expressed in cell membrane→ therefore, adsorbs RBCs onto surface

PARAMYXOVIRUS

(parainfluenza types 1 and 3)

- parainfluenza virus (PIV) infects respiratory epithelial cells→spread from cell to cell within nose and pharynx
- after 1st replication→nasal congestion and pharyngitis→spreads to larynx and tracheal epithelial cells→croup (fusion of cells cause decreased beating of respiratory cilia)
- immune system resolves infection; but immunity does not last

Epidemiology

- spreads by respiratory droplets; person-to-person; virus shed for 7–10 days during active infection
- PIV 1 and 2→croup in 2–5 year olds
- PIV 3→bronchiolitis and pneumonia in <1 year old
- PIV 4→colds in all ages

Clinical Diseases

- *croup:* appearance of seal-bark cough
- *bronchiolitis:* can progress to pneumonia

Diagnosis

detection of PIV antigen; hemadsorption with guinea pig RBCs; isolate identified by hemagglutination inhibition

Treatment

supportive; nebulized cool mist and maintain upper airway

RUBULAVIRUS

(PIV 2, 4a, 4b, mumps virus)

- genome encodes 7 proteins; nucleocapsid has NP, L, P; envelope→HN and F

Pathogenesis

- mumps start in upper respiratory tract→ replicate in mucosal epithelial cells and local lymphocytes→viremia to target tissue (salivary glands, CNS, testes, ovaries, mammary glands, myocardium, and pancreas)→ hallmark is swelling due to parotitis

Epidemiology

- mumps human disease spread by saliva; contagion precedes symptoms; not teratogenic

Clinical Diseases

- *mumps:* prodrome→"earache" from swollen parotid gland→both glands swell (2nd may lag behind a few days)→fever falls when swelling greatest (Wharton's and Stenson's ducts swell and hemorrhage)
- **epididymo-orchitis:** testicles swell
- meningitis
- **other complications:** encephalitis; pancreatitis; neurosensory deafness; mastitis, arthritis, myocarditis, nephritis, oophoritis

Diagnosis

made clinically; IgM antibody to NP protein; culture of blood, CSF, saliva, or urine

Treatment

none; vaccine

MORBILLIVIRUS

- measles virus
- envelope contains protein F and HA hemagglutinin; no neuraminidase

Pathogenesis

- respiratory cells infected first→to lymph nodes →2nd replication→viremia→ secondary lymph organs→replication→ 2nd viremia→many tissues
- viremia continues until rash begins; viruria continues for several days after it ends
- form syncytia (multinucleated giant cells); cytoplasmic inclusions can be seen in infected cells; cell lysis except in brain (persistent infection)
- rash caused by CTL attack on infected endothelial cells of the small blood vessels and capillaries

Complications

- secondary bacterial infection common
- malnourished patients: decreases intestinal absorption, decreases hepatic vitamin A stores, children suffer corneal xerophthalmia (corneal ulceration and blindness)
- children with deficiency of T-cells: atypical measles→giant cell pneumonia without rash; infection of macrophages→ decreased function (virus binds CD46→decreases IL-12→T-cell anergy)
- CNS disease: acute postinfectious measles encephalitis (autoimmune demyelination); subacute measles encephalitis; subacute sclerosing panencephalitis (SSPE)→years later; limited replication of virus in brain leads to death

Epidemiology

- cyclic epidemics (every 2–3 years)
- highly contagious; transmission by respiratory droplets

Clinical Diseases

- **measles:** high fever, conjunctivitis (photophobia), coryza (acute rhinitis), and cough (most infectious stage)→**Koplik's spots** (white nodules most commonly occurring on the buccal mucosa)→ maculopapular exanthem (starts below ears and spreads to rest of face)→body rash
- **bronchiolitis, laryngitis, tracheobronchitis, pneumonia:** older patients and children with deficiency of T-cells
- encephalitis
- *SSPE*: 5–7 years after infection→ myoclonus, personality changes, focal neurologic deficits→paralysis→coma and death

Diagnosis

detection of measles antigen; giant cells and nuclear inclusions; serology; SSPE→presence of antibody in CSF

Treatment

none; vaccine

PNEUMOVIRUS

(respiratory syncytial virus→RSV)

- no HA or neuraminidase; attachment to protein G
- MOST FREQUENT CAUSE OF FATAL RESPIRATORY INFECTION AMONG INFANTS

Pathogenesis

- localized respiratory tract infection with syncytia; infects epithelial cells and macrophages; no dissemination; travels down to bronchioles and lower lung→atelectasis and bronchiolar obstruction
- pathology caused by viral infection and CMI; necrosis of bronchi obstructs airways; natural immunity does not prevent reinfection

Epidemiology

- infection symptomatic with lower respiratory tract infection
- very contagious; shed for weeks; transmitted on hands, fomites, respiratory droplets; can survive in respiratory secretions on skin or surfaces for 30 minutes

Clinical Syndromes

- **respiratory diseases** (from colds to pneumonia); older children and adults→rhinorrhea; children→febrile colds, rhinitis, pharyngitis
- **bronchiolitis and/or pneumonia** in children <1 year.

Diagnosis

RSV antigen detection

Treatment

respiratory isolation to prevent spread; supportive care to prevent anoxia; treatment with nebulized ribavirin to decrease severity and duration

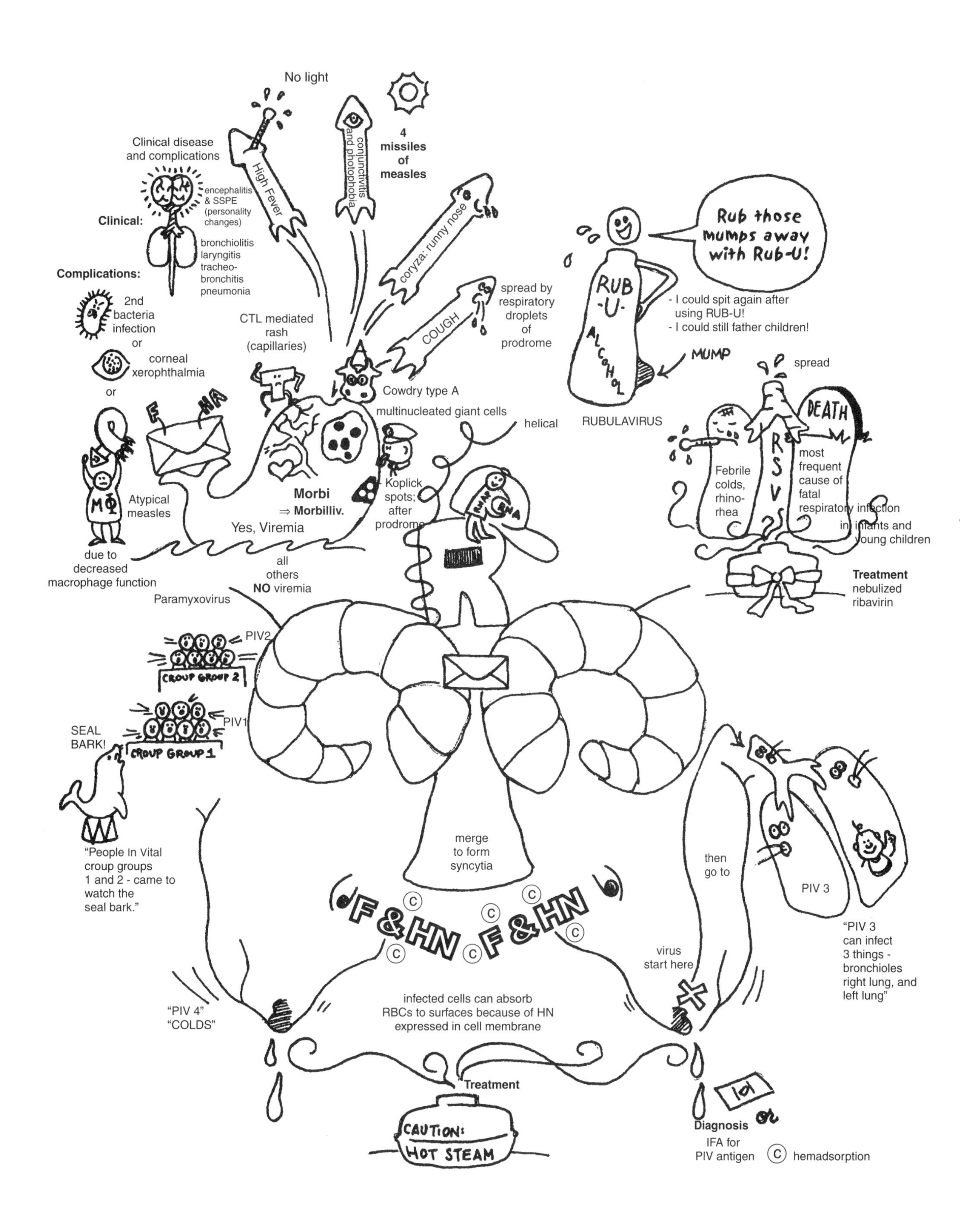
No light
4 missiles of measles
High Fever
conjunctivitis and photophobia
coryza: runny nose
COUGH
spread by respiratory droplets of prodrome
Clinical disease and complications
Clinical:
encephalitis & SSPE (personality changes)
bronchiolitis laryngitis tracheo-bronchitis pneumonia
Complications:
2nd bacteria infection
or
corneal xerophthalmia
or
CTL mediated rash (capillaries)
Cowdry type A
multinucleated giant cells
helical
F
HA
MΦ
Atypical measles
due to decreased macrophage function
Morbi ⇒ Morbilliv.
Yes, Viremia
Koplick spots; after prodrome
all others NO viremia
Paramyxovirus
Rub those mumps away with Rub-U!
RUB -U-
ALCOHOL
MUMP
- I could spit again after using RUB-U!
- I could still father children!
RUBULAVIRUS
spread
DEATH
RSV
Febrile colds, rhino-rhea
most frequent cause of fatal respiratory infection in infants and young children
Treatment nebulized ribavirin
PIV2
CROUP GROUP 2
PIV1
CROUP GROUP 1
SEAL BARK!
"People In Vital croup groups 1 and 2 - came to watch the seal bark."
merge to form syncytia
F & HN
F & HN
"PIV 4" "COLDS"
infected cells can absorb RBCs to surfaces because of HN expressed in cell membrane
then go to
virus start here
PIV 3
"PIV 3 can infect 3 things - bronchioles right lung, and left lung"
Treatment
CAUTION: HOT STEAM
Diagnosis
IFA for PIV antigen
or
hemadsorption

NOTES

RHABDOVIRIDAE

- genera that infect humans: vesiculovirus—vesicular stomatitis viruses (VSV); Lyssavirus—rabies virus, Duvenhage virus, Lagos bat virus, Mokola virus
- bullet-shaped, enveloped (contains G glycoprotein→viral attachment protein; envelope lined with matrix protein (M)→maintain virus shape; helical nucleocapsid and transcriptase

Replication

- G proteins attach to CSR→internalized by endocytosis→replicates in cytoplasm→producing inclusion bodies (Negri bodies)→released by budding through plasma membrane
- except for rabies virus→cell death and lysis are outcome of infection

Pathogenesis and Immunity

- infection from bite of rabid animal→G-protein binds to nicotinic Ach receptors on muscle cells→replication→migration to NMJ→replicates in neuronal cells→to DRG to spinal cord to brain (ascending infection)→dissemination to richly innervated areas (descending infection)→little immune response (if type IV hypersensitivity response occurs death comes more quickly)→once clinical disease occurs death is imminent
- factors of incubation period: inoculum, closeness of wound to brain, age, and immune status; limbic system infection early→increasing cortisol production leading to classic aggressive behavior; later cortical system leading to coma and respiratory arrest

Epidemiology

- transmitted by bite or scratch (mostly dogs and bats (USA)
- classic zoonotic infection→animal to human
- dog principal reservoir, vaccination in US has reduced spread to the sylvatic type (wild animals infecting domestic animals)
- vesicular stomatitis→disease in cattle and spread to humans via bite of blackflies, mites, mosquitoes, or sandflies

Clinical Diseases

- rabies: incubation period can last up to a year; prodrome→neurological symptoms
- furious rabies: **hydrophobia (painful spasms of inspiratory and laryngeal muscles at the sound, smell, touch, or thought of water),** aggression, seizures, etc.; seizures can cause cardiac arrest because of increased heart rate; saliva production increases; death within 7 days
- paralytic or dumb rabies; paresthesia progresses to paralysis of limbs and then to fatal paralysis (respiratory arrest)
- once symptoms begin death inevitable
- vesicular stomatitis: vesicular lesions in mouth, diarrhea, etc. resolves within 10 days
- Duvenhage virus, Lagos bat virus, and Mokola virus cause rabies-like neurologic disease

Diagnosis

brain examination of offending animal for Negri bodies; **evidence of infection in victim, including symptoms and detection of antibody, occur too late for intervention→treatment should begin as soon as exposure is suspected**

Treatment

prevention only hope to save victim; initiate therapy unless animal is tested not rabid; cleanse wound with substance that would inactivate the virus; irrigate wound with human rabies Ig (HRIG); administer one dose of HRIG; immunize; pre-exposure vaccination; prevention by vaccination of animals

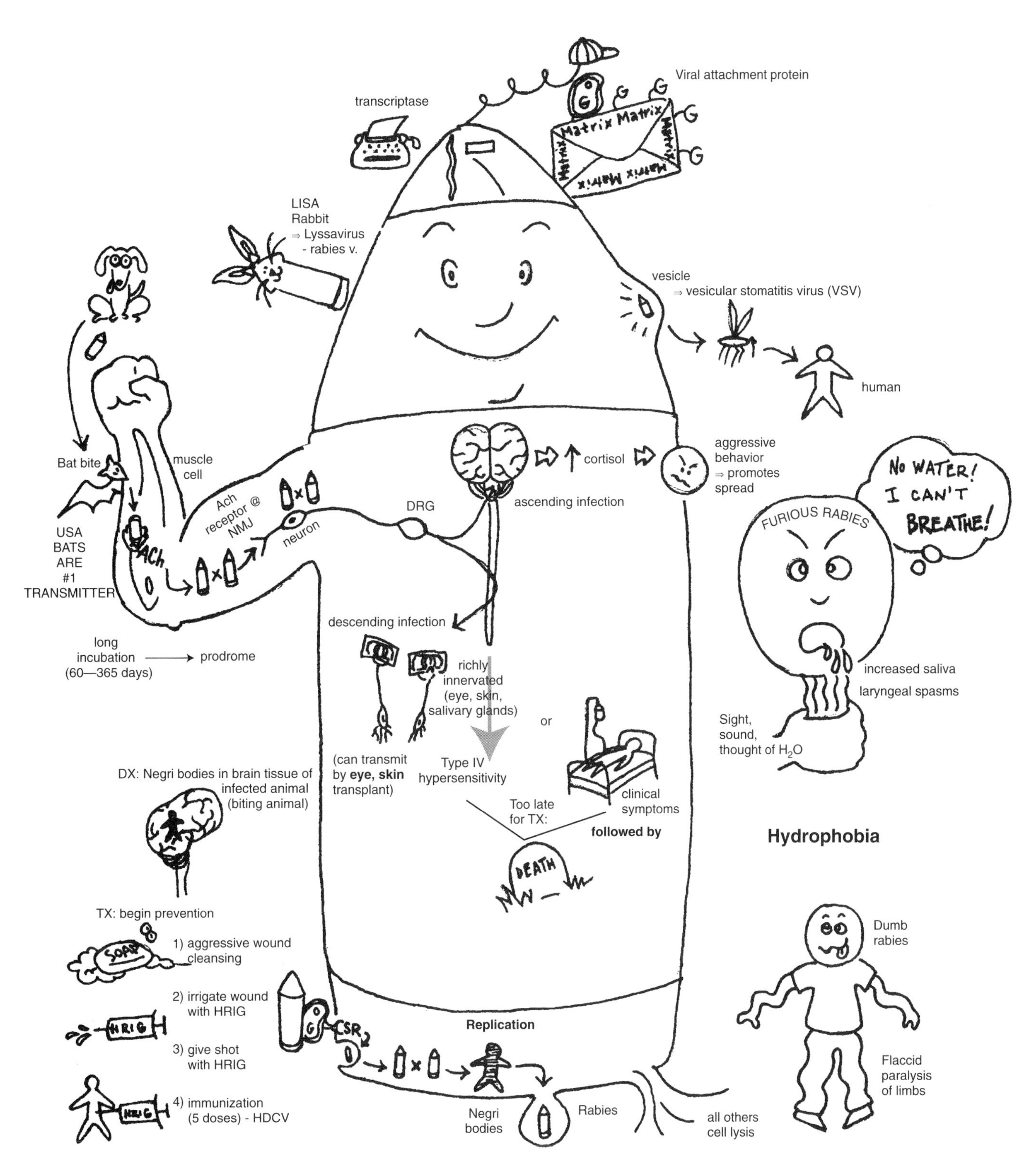
Viral attachment protein
transcriptase
Matrix Matrix
LISA
Rabbit
⇒ Lyssavirus
- rabies v.
vesicle
⇒ vesicular stomatitis virus (VSV)
human
Bat bite
muscle
cell
Ach
receptor @
NMJ
neuron
DRG
cortisol
ascending infection
aggressive
behavior
⇒ promotes
spread
USA
BATS
ARE
#1
TRANSMITTER
NO WATER!
I CAN'T
BREATHE!
FURIOUS RABIES
descending infection
long
incubation
(60—365 days)
prodrome
richly
innervated
(eye, skin,
salivary glands)
or
increased saliva
laryngeal spasms
Sight,
sound,
thought of H_2O
DX: Negri bodies in brain tissue of
infected animal
(biting animal)
(can transmit
by eye, skin
transplant)
Type IV
hypersensitivity
Too late
for TX:
clinical
symptoms
followed by
DEATH
Hydrophobia
TX: begin prevention
SOAP
1) aggressive wound
cleansing
2) irrigate wound
with HRIG
HRIG
3) give shot
with HRIG
4) immunization
(5 doses) - HDCV
Replication
CSR
Negri
bodies
Rabies
all others
cell lysis
Dumb
rabies
Flaccid
paralysis
of limbs
prevention: vaccinate domestic pets

NOTES

BUNYAVIRIDAE

- arbothropod-borne: bunyavirus, phlebovirus, nairovirus
- rodent spread: hantavirus
- enveloped; 3 helical nucleocapsids; **NO MATRIX PROTEIN**; RNA segments: L (large), M (medium), S (small, some genera ambisense)

Pathogenesis

- inoculation→viremia→replication→2nd viremia→target tissue (CNS, liver, kidney, vascular endothelium); hantavirus stays in lungs

Epidemiology

- need for specific vector confined to geographical location
- hantavirus inhalation of aerosolized rodent urine or rodent contact spreads disease to humans

Clinical Syndromes

- California encephalitis: La Crosse virus; occurs after 2nd viremia
- Crimean-Congo hemorrhagic fever: sudden onset; fever and sharp back pain followed by pulmonary edema and shock
- hemorrhagic fever with renal syndrome: proteinuria followed by petechiae, GI bleeding, hemorrhagic pneumonia→during recovery renal tubular disease with oliguria
- hantavirus pulmonary syndrome: adult respiratory distress syndrome; Muerto Canyon fever, flu-like symptoms followed by interstitial pulmonary edema
- oropouche fever, mild; all recover
- Rift Valley fever, bite of sandfly→fever, headache, etc.→3 courses: mild encephalitis; retinitis and loss of central vision; hemorrhagic fever
- sandfly fever: self-limiting dengue- like syndrome

Diagnosis

culture and identification

Treatment

none; interruption of transmission best prevention

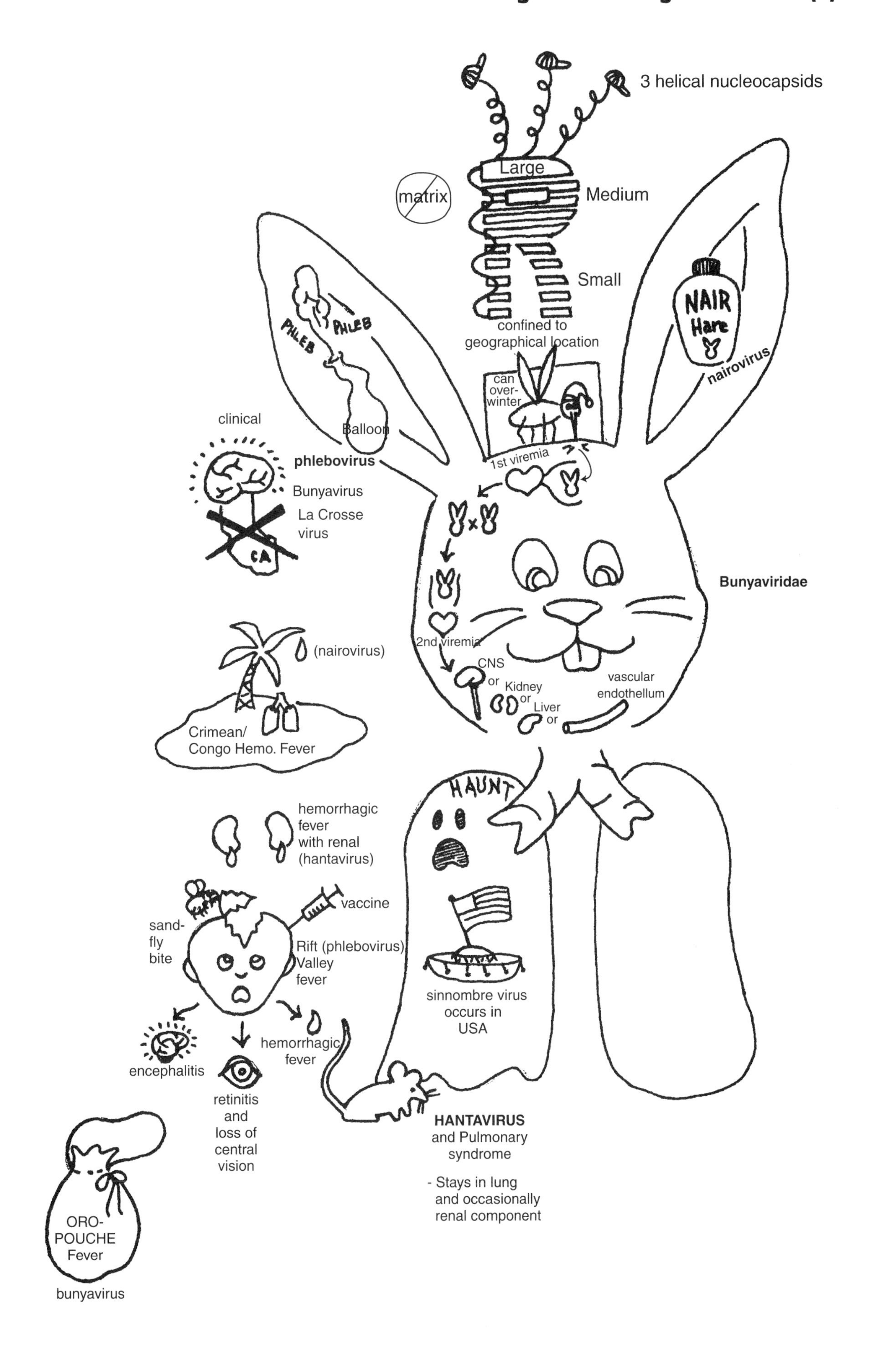
3 helical nucleocapsids
matrix
Large
Medium
Small
confined to
geographical location
can
over-
winter
NAIR
Hare
nairovirus
clinical
Balloon
PHLEB
PHLEB
phlebovirus
1st viremia
Bunyavirus
La Crosse
virus
CA
Bunyaviridae
(nairovirus)
2nd viremia
CNS
or
Kidney
or
Liver
or
vascular
endothellum
Crimean/
Congo Hemo. Fever
HAUNT
hemorrhagic
fever
with renal
(hantavirus)
vaccine
sand-
fly
bite
Rift (phlebovirus)
Valley
fever
sinnombre virus
occurs in
USA
encephalitis
hemorrhagic
fever
retinitis
and
loss of
central
vision
HANTAVIRUS
and Pulmonary
syndrome
- Stays in lung
and occasionally
renal component
ORO-
POUCHE
Fever
bunyavirus

NOTES

FILOVIRIDAE

- Marburg virus, Ebola virus, and Reston virus
- infectious monkeys pass to humans
- filamentous, enveloped; encode 7 proteins
- enters host cell via phagocytosis; replicates in cytoplasm; produces elongated inclusion bodies; virus escapes by budding through plasma membrane

Pathogenesis

- replication in adrenal glands, kidney, liver, and spleen cause alteration in endothelial arachidonate metabolism→tissue necrosis
- early leukopenia then neutrophilia; hemorrhage leads to edema and hypovolemic shock
- **BIOSAFETY LEVEL 4 organisms considered extremely dangerous**

Epidemiology

- Ebola risk factors: contaminated needles, caring for Ebola patients, preparation of Ebola victims for burial, sexual contact with infectious individual; possible respiratory transmission
- antigenic variation and increase/decrease of virulence

Clinical Diseases

- Ebola virus: causes most severe hemorrhagic disease known; sudden onset of arthralgia, fever, etc.→2nd or 3rd day: sore throat, difficulty swallowing, vomiting, and abdominal pain→5th day profuse bleeding from mucous membranes followed by death
- Marburg virus: similar to Ebola with lower death rate

Diagnosis

use **EXTREME CAUTION** in specimen handling; culture body fluids; detection of large eosinophilic cytoplasmic inclusions

Treatment

supportive; **STRICT ISOLATION and BARRIER PROTOCOL**

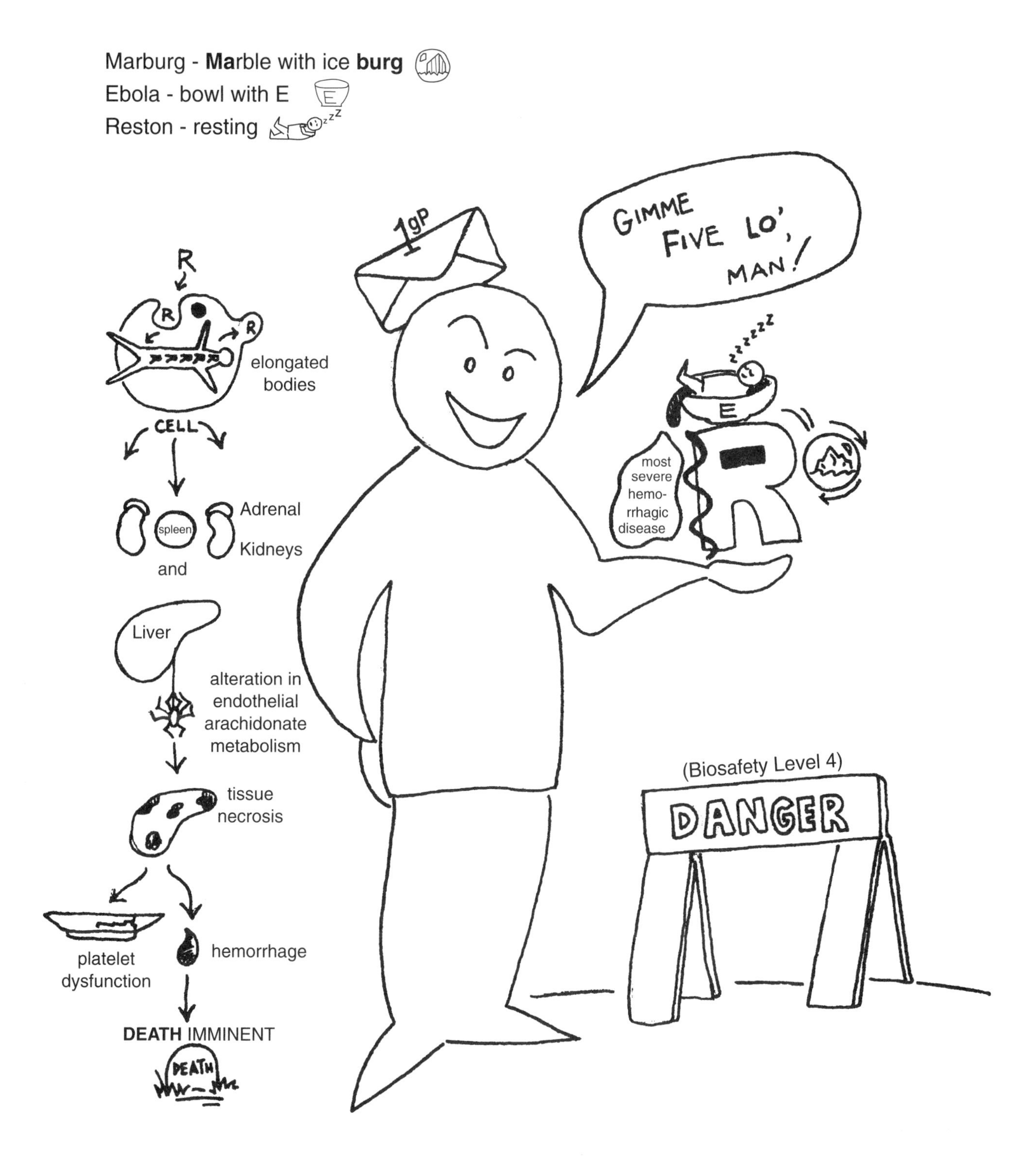
Marburg - Marble with ice burg
Ebola - bowl with E
Reston - resting
GIMME FIVE LO', MAN!
1gP
R
R
R
elongated bodies
CELL
spleen
Adrenal
Kidneys
and
Liver
alteration in endothelial arachidonate metabolism
tissue necrosis
platelet dysfunction
hemorrhage
DEATH IMMINENT
DEATH
E
most severe hemo-rrhagic disease
(Biosafety Level 4)
DANGER

ARENAVIRIDAE

- two serogroups: LCM-LAS complex (lymphocytic choriomeningitis [LCM] and Lassa virus); Tacaribe complex: 1) Flexal, Parana, Pichinde, and Tamiami, 2) Ampari, Guanarito, Junin, Machupo, Sabia, Tacaribe (non-infectious to humans), 3) Latino and Oliveros
- capsids enclose cellular ribosomes→ particles appear full of sand; circular envelope; contain 2 helical nucleocapsid segments and transcriptase; RNA circularized
- most of segment (–) but portion of it is (+)→ambisense; replicate in cytoplasm and viruses bud through plasma membrane

Pathogenesis

- LCM infection is immune-mediated because only develop meningitis when CTLs attack virus in brain cells
- antibodies protect against Junin and Machupo; CMI involved in resolution of Lassa fever
- in Lassa fever bleeding caused by platelet dysfunction

Epidemiology

- infects specific rodents and virus confined to rodent's habitat; shedding in rodent saliva, urine, and feces
- **Lassa and Tacaribe viruses are BIOSAFETY LEVEL 4**

Clinical Diseases

- lymphatic choriomeningitis: majority asymptomatic; for those who do show symptoms, recovery is slow but usually complete
- Lassa fever—gradual onset of fever→ cough and lumbar and joint pain→frontal headache→tender abdomen; life-threatening→facial and neck edema from capillary leakage, **damage to 8th cranial nerve**→hearing loss; transmitted in utero and breast milk
- hemorrhagic fever: Argentinian, Bolivian, and Venezuelan; acute neurologic disease or pulmonary edema can occur; hypotension usual cause of death

Diagnosis

use **EXTREME CAUTION** when handling specimens

Treatment

strict isolation; management of hypotensive shock; Lassa fever can be treated with IV ribavirin during first 6 days; Argentinian hemorrhagic fever treat with high titer convalescent plasma

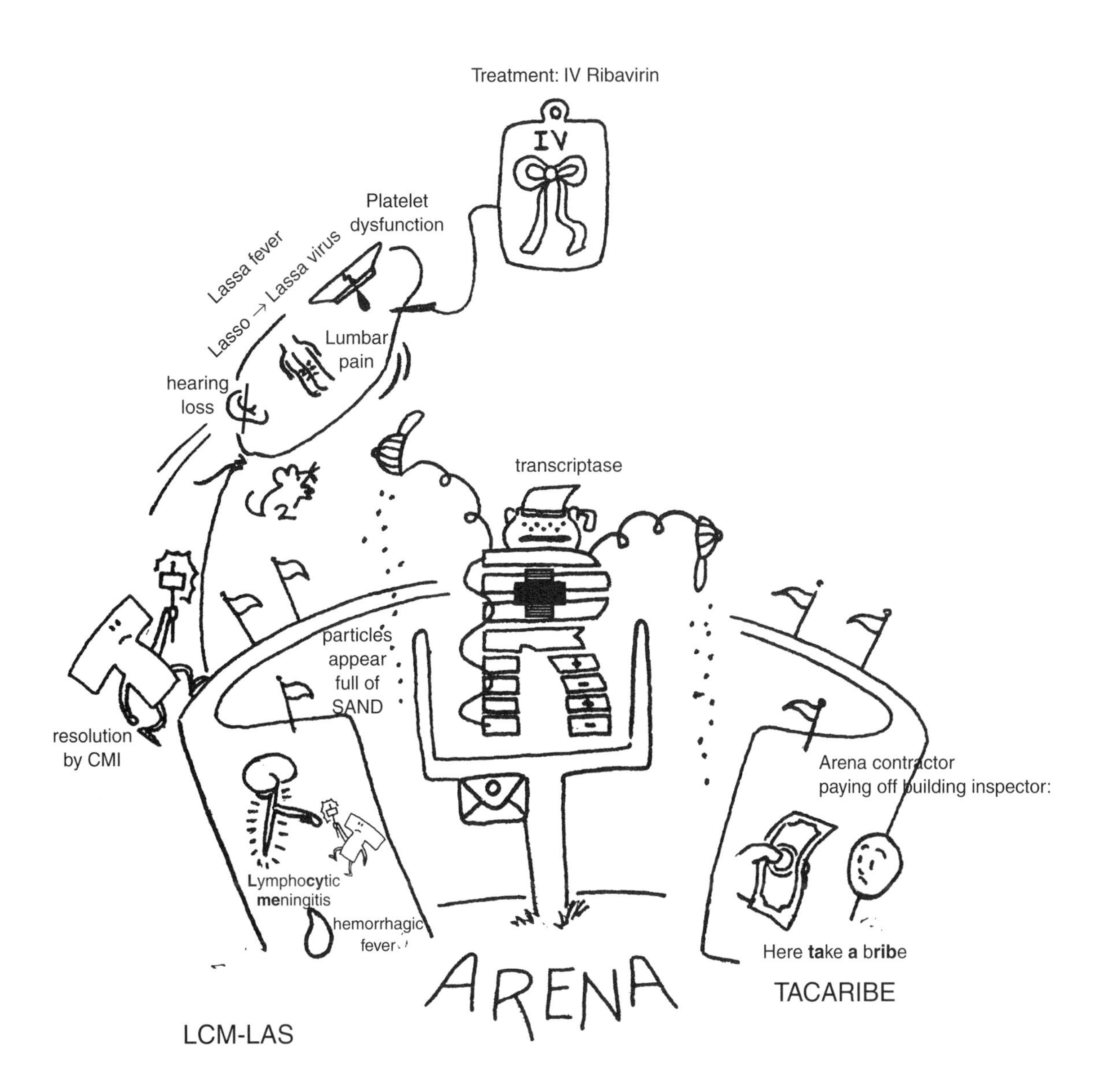
Treatment: IV Ribavirin
IV
Platelet dysfunction
Lassa fever
Lasso → Lassa virus
Lumbar pain
hearing loss
transcriptase
particles appear full of SAND
resolution by CMI
Lymphocytic meningitis
hemorrhagic fever
Arena contractor paying off building inspector:
Here take a bribe
ARENA
TACARIBE
LCM-LAS

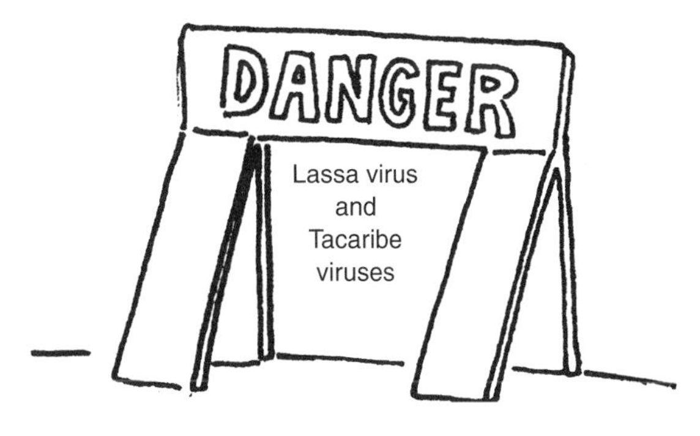
DANGER
Lassa virus and Tacaribe viruses

NOTES

REOVIRIDAE

⇒ double stuffed **OREO** ⇒ ds RNA

- rotavirus, coltivirus, orbivirus, orthoreovirus
- nonenveloped, icosahedral; two concentric capsids surround core of 10–12 segments of double-stranded RNA; contains RNAP; mRNA cap; resistant to low pH, heat, and proteolysis

Replication

- rotavirus ingestion→replication in intestine→cleavage of capsid by intestinal trypsin→activates virus into **infectious subviral particle (ISP)** by cleaving viral attachment proteins→ISP enters cell by viropexis→partially uncoated→escapes to cytosol→macromolecules enter and leave viral core where 11 dsRNA segments are maintained **(parental RNA always remains in core)**→viral RNAP transcribes (–) RNA to mRNA and capped→mRNA leave core→translated in cytoplasm→viral proteins and mRNAs assembled into core-like structures→(+) strand in core copied to produce (–)→(+) and (–) associate as progeny dsRNA→virions accumulate until cell lyses

ROTAVIRUS

- human pathogenic in groups A, B, C

Pathogenesis and Immunity

- resistant to stomach acid
- cause blunting of intestinal microvilli; infiltrate seen in lamina propria but no inflammation; causes carbohydrate malabsorption, and water loss with ion loss; severe dehydration follows

Epidemiology

- occur most frequently in children (6–24 months); shedding of virus occurs after diarrhea starts
- immunity requires secretory IgA; neither active nor passive antibody from mother to neonate offers protection: neonates are asymptomatic because they lack proteases and adults have less severe disease because they lack receptor

Clinical Disease

- incubation followed by watery diarrhea; dehydration greatest threat

Diagnosis

EIA to detect viral antigen in stool or EM for viral particles

Treatment

no antiviral therapy; supportive care

COLTIVIRUS

- 12 dsRNA segments
- **Colorado tick fever virus and Eyach virus**

Pathogenesis

- Colorado tick fever infects erythroid precursor cells without damage; continues to replicate; persistent viremia; causes serious hemorrhagic disease if virus infects vascular endothelial cells and smooth muscle cells

Epidemiology

- reservoir→golden-mantled ground squirrel; vector→wood tick

Clinical Disease

- Colorado tick fever—acute disease resembles dengue
- disease biphasic—2 phases of leukopenia and thrombocytopenia with gradual remission after 2nd; lasting immunity occurs
- hemorrhage or meningitis—children

Diagnosis

detection of viral antigens

Treatment

supportive

REOVIRUS AND ORBIVIRUS

Reovirus

no significant pathology

Orbivirus

mainly animal pathogens (blue tongue virus); Kemerovo virus causes meningitis

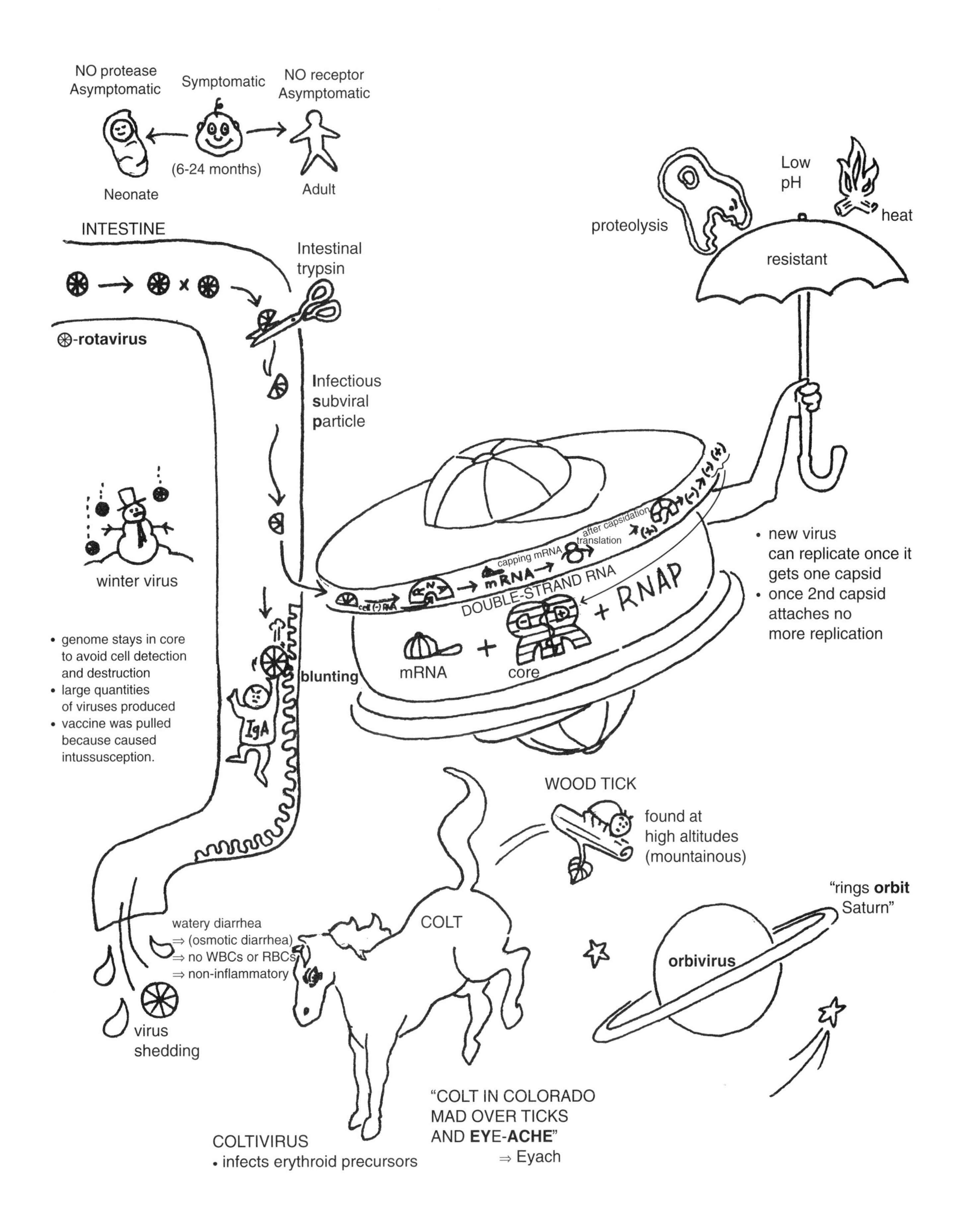
NO protease
Asymptomatic
Symptomatic
NO receptor
Asymptomatic
(6-24 months)
Neonate
Adult
INTESTINE
Intestinal
trypsin
-rotavirus
Infectious
subviral
particle
winter virus
• genome stays in core to avoid cell detection and destruction
• large quantities of viruses produced
• vaccine was pulled because caused intussusception.
blunting
IgA
proteolysis
Low
pH
heat
resistant
capping mRNA
after capsidation
translation
mRNA
DOUBLE-STRAND RNA
+ RNAP
mRNA
core
• new virus can replicate once it gets one capsid
• once 2nd capsid attaches no more replication
WOOD TICK
found at
high altitudes
(mountainous)
"rings orbit
Saturn"
orbivirus
COLT
watery diarrhea
⇒ (osmotic diarrhea)
⇒ no WBCs or RBCs
⇒ non-inflammatory
virus
shedding
"COLT IN COLORADO
MAD OVER TICKS
AND EYE-ACHE"
⇒ Eyach
COLTIVIRUS
• infects erythroid precursors

NOTES

RETROVIRIDAE

- enveloped diploid single-stranded (+)RNA
- **oncornavirinae:** immortalize target cells; cause human T-cell leukemia or lymphoma, tropical spastic paraparesis; possibly hairy cell leukemia
- **lentivirinae:** slow viruses that cause immunosuppressive and/or neurological disease; cause AIDS
- **spumavirinae:** produce a distinct foamy cytopathic effect in cells but have not been associated with clinical disease
- endogenous retroviruses: vertically transmitted; integrated in host without lytic cycle

Structure

- spherical particles
- capsid contains genome: two identical (+)RNA, reverse transcriptase (RT), integrase (IN), two cellular tRNAs (that serve as primers for replication)
- each linear haploid genome segment has 5′ cap and 3′ polyA tail
- genome contains 3 major genes that encode for: gag—group specific antigen; core and capsid proteins; pol—RT, protease, and integrase; sometimes the protease is a separate gene (pro); env—envelope glycoproteins
- long terminal repeat (LTR) sequences at end of each genome; carry promoter, enhancer, sequences for binding regulatory proteins; allow to integrate into chromosome

Replication

- attachment of glycoprotein spikes to CSR→enter cell by fusion or endocytosis→core proteins and genome are released into cytoplasm→RT synthesizes (–) DNA complementary from (+) RNA genome→then dsDNA→U3 and U5 (at the end of viral DNA) are duplicated→producing LTRs→enters cell nucleus→IN catalyzes integration of viral genome into host→now provirus and under cellular control→cellular transcription produces mRNAs or full-length (+) RNA for new virions
- replication depends on: ability of host cell to use LTR sequences; other agents that induce transcription including other viral infections, and any encoded viral oncogenes that promote cell growth
- gag, gag-pol, and env mRNAs must be cleaved by viral protease to become functional
- immature and noninfectious virion: 2 copies genome, +2 tRNAs bud through plasma membrane
- protease cleavage produces infectious virions

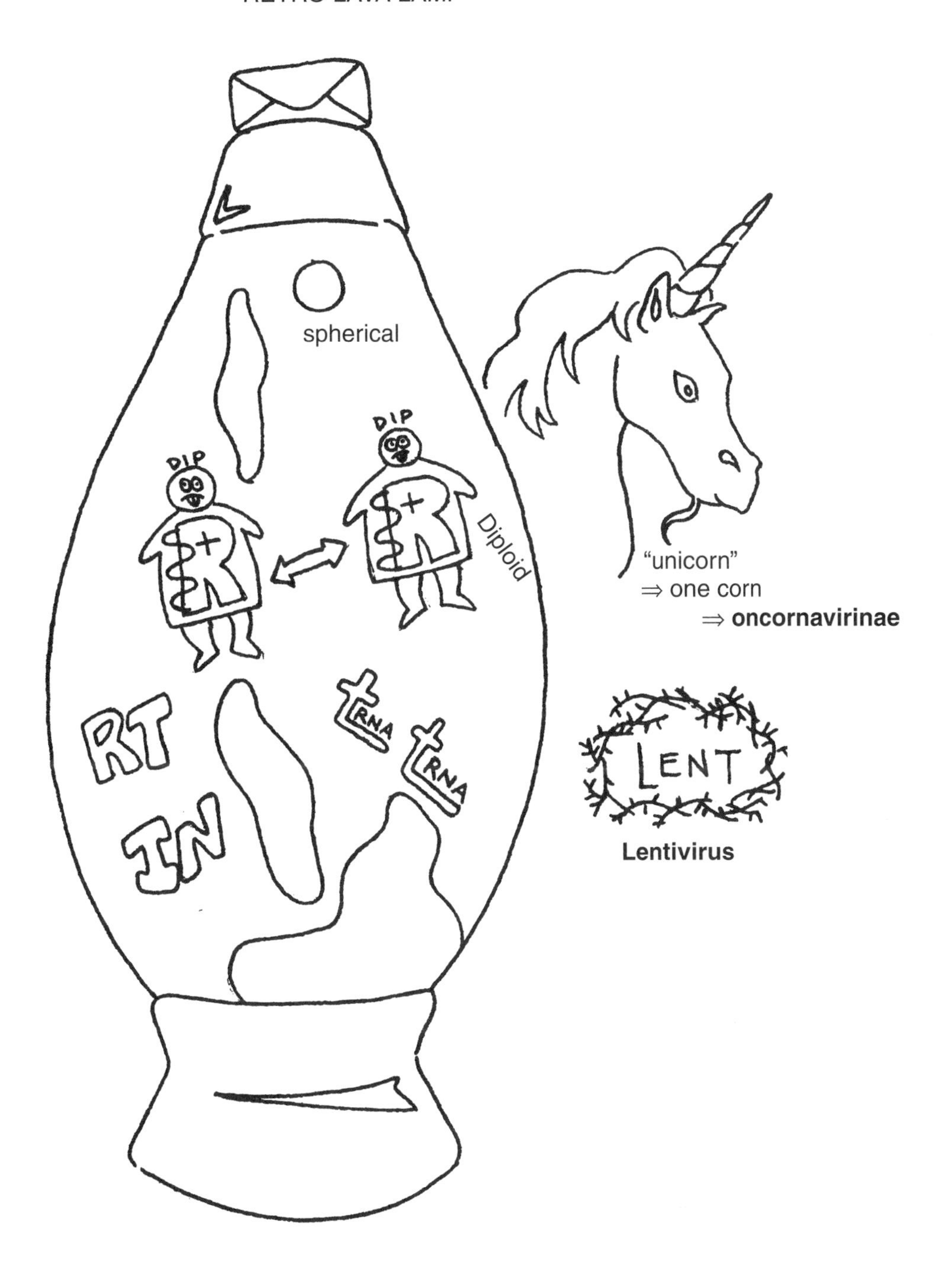
RETRO LAVA LAMP
spherical
DIP
DIP
Diploid
RT
IN
tRNA
tRNA
"unicorn"
⇒ one corn
⇒ **oncornavirinae**
LENT
Lentivirus

ONCOVIRINAE

⇒ one unicorn

- carcinoma: solid tumor of epithelial origin
- leukemia: cancer of circulation—leukocytes
- lymphoma: solid tumor of lymphoctye origin
- sarcoma: solid tumor of mesenchymal origin

NOTES

VIRUSES ASSOCIATED WITH ONCOGENESIS

DNA Viruses

- Epstein-Barr virus: Burkitt's lymphoma; nasopharyngeal carcinoma
- HBV: primary hepatocellular carcinoma
- human herpesvirus 8: Kaposi's sarcoma; non-Hodgkin's lymphoma
- HPV: cervical and anogenital carcinoma; squamous cell carcinoma

RNA Viruses

- HCV: primary hepatocellular carcinoma
- human T-cell lymphotropic virus (HTLV); adult T-cell leukemia or lymphoma

VIRAL ONCOGENIC PROCESSES

DNA Viruses

- in non-permissive cells the viral genome transforms the cell; genome in one of 2 forms: integrated or episomal

RNA Viruses

- always integrate into host genome; produce progeny and cell transformation; carry viral oncogenes (*v-onc*)

Cellular Mechanisms of Growth Control

- **proto-oncogenes (*c-onc*):** induce cell transformation including growth factors, growth factor receptors, intracellular signal transducers, nuclear transcription factors
- **tumor suppressor genes: *p53* and *RB* (retinoblastoma);** block cell transformation

Mechanisms of Viral Transformation and Oncogenesis

- introduction of *v-onc* gene→cells multiply without restraint
- virus integration upstream from *c-onc* gene (removal of down-regulation function)→ cells multiply without restraint
- *c-onc* comes under control of strong promoter
- virus produces *trans*-activating factor for *c-onc* gene
- *c-onc* gene becomes "locked on" during mutation
- viral proteins inactivate tumor suppressor gene products

Total Oncogenic Process

- multistage process; tumor must evade immune control, metastasize, become independent of tissue growth factors, establish blood supply, avoid apoptosis

Categories of Oncoviruses

- exogenous viruses: spread horizontally; rapid (acute): carry *v-onc*, death in short time; or slow: no *onc* present (known human oncovirus)
- endogenous viruses: previously silent integrated viral genomes are expressed due to induction by irradiation, etc.; vertically transmitted; usually not pathogenic
- replication competent virus vs. replication defective (addition of *v-onc* gene stops vital viral protein expression)

Human *c-onc* Gene and Associated Disease

- *c-abl*→chronic myelogenous leukemia
- *c-fos*→human T-cell leukemia or lymphoma
- *c-ras*→bladder carcinoma
- *c-myc*→Burkitt's lymphoma; small cell lung carcinoma; breast cancer
- *c-erbB*→squamous cell carcinoma; glioblastoma
- *c-sis*→human T-cell leukemia or lymphoma

Human T-cell Lymphotropic Viruses (HTLVs)

- infectious CD4+ cells
- **do not contain *v-onc* genes but carry 2 regulatory genes:**
- *HTLV-I*→adult T-cell leukemia or lymphoma (ATLL)
- *HTLV-II*→hairy cell leukemia

Pathogenesis

- integrated; regulatory proteins (tax and rex) essential for replication
- tax promotes transcription of host cellular genes including IL-2 and IL-2 receptor gene→proliferation of T-cells; up-regulates transcription of *c-fos* and platelet-derived growth factor gene; *trans*-activator that affects many other cells
- rex regulates splicing of mRNA, promotes production of progeny; inhibits own gene and tax; responsible for periods of latency and production

Epidemiology

- transmission: vertical (mother to infant); horizontally through sexual intercourse or blood contact

Diseases

- ATLL: develops 20–40 years post infection; acute leads to death in <1 year; bone lesions, etc.
- tropical spastic paraparesis: progressive demyelinating disease; infects long motor nerves of spinal cord; lower body weakness; resembles MS but does not remit; mental abilities and cranial nerves remain intact

Diagnosis

Antibody detection; transformed CD4+ cells have a pleomorphic lobular appearance and contain large convoluted nuclei

Treatment

ATLL is fatal; prevention—screening blood supply and safe sex

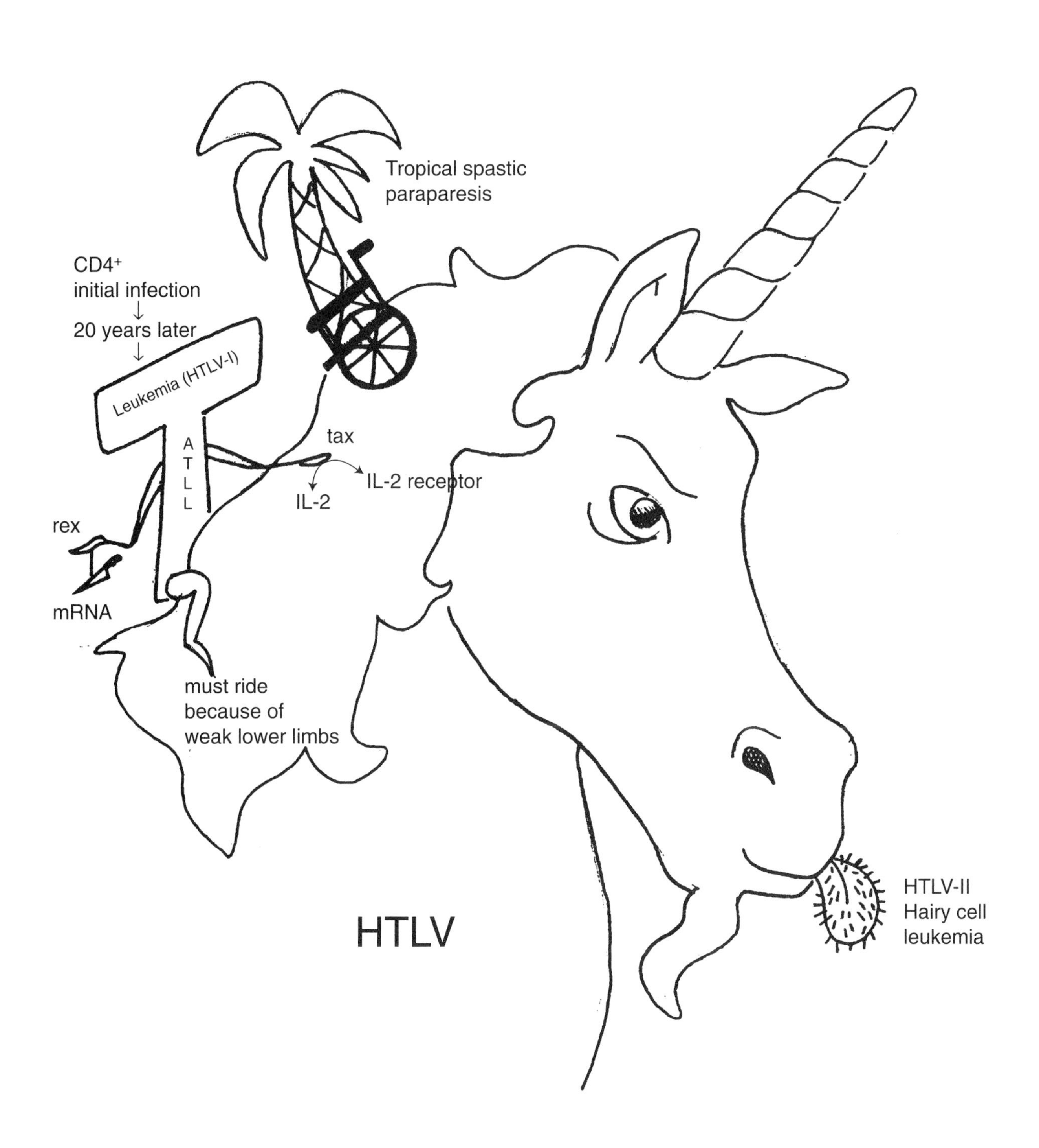
Tropical spastic paraparesis
CD4+
initial infection
↓
20 years later
↓
Leukemia (HTLV-I)
ATLL
tax
IL-2
IL-2 receptor
rex
mRNA
must ride because of weak lower limbs
HTLV-II Hairy cell leukemia
HTLV

LENTIVIRINAE

- type D morphology
- HIV
- diseases have long periods of latent infection followed by neurological and/or immunological disease

HUMAN IMMUNODEFICIENCY VIRUS (HIV)

- spherical, enveloped with cone-shaped core
- envelope products are glycoproteins: gp120 (primary adhesin molecule); gp41 (fusion protein)
- gag products: p16/17 (viral matrix protein); p24/25 (capsid protein)
- core: 2 copies ss(+) RNA, 2 cellular tRNAs (captured during budding), pol enzymes: RT, IN, PR (protease)
- HIV-1 genome: 9 proteins and 8 additional structural proteins from protease cleavage

Replication

- same as other retroviruses; unless cell is activated the provirus remains latent→ RNAP II is required for transcription which is only present in actively replicating cells
- activating agents: cytokines, mitogens, cellular stress factors, and heterologous viruses (CMV, HSV, HBV, and HTLV)→all induce release of NF-κB from its inhibitor, I-κB→NF-κB enhancer elements in LTR→3 classes mRNA produced (alternate splicing produces more)

Replication Control (by 3 Proteins)

- **Tat:** binds to TAR (*trans*-activating response) region; prevents premature termination of transcription; required for significant levels of HIV mRNA to be produced
- **Rev:** binds to Rev response region within envelope gene of mRNA and transports them to cytoplasm for translation
- **Nef:** essential for the replication of HIV within macrophages and monocytes→ relates to down-regulation of CD4 and IL-2 expression

Pathogenesis

- loss of immune responsiveness (immunosuppression); depletion of CD4+ T lymphocytes
- AIDS precipitated by HIV-1and individual becomes susceptible to opportunistic infection (CD4+ T cell <400/μm; HIV neurologic disease; intractable diarrhea)
- viral tropism: CD4+ T-cells; CD4 – T-cells (bowel and renal); brain astrocytes and oligodendrocytes
- infection of CD4+ cell: attachment via gp120 and co-receptor→cellular CD26 cleaves V# loop of gp120→exposes fusogenic domain of gp41→membrane fusion→liberation of core into cytosol

Origin and Genetics

- HIV-1 evolved from simian immunodeficiency virus; 5 major genotypic subtypes or clades; HIV-2 45% identical to type 1

Modes of Transmission

- sexual intercourse; if penetrating partner has STD the risk of transmission is greater due to the presence of more leukocytes; if receptive partner has STD lesions of genitourinary mucosa transmission enhanced because resistant barrier removed; male more likely to transmit to female
- blood and blood products; sharing needle and syringes
- perinatal: via amniotic fluid, blood, or genital secretions, transplacentally and breast feeding

Origin of Immunosuppression

- CD4+ cells depleted: direct—HIV cytolytic; indirect—immune processes result in cell destruction
- factors responsible for immunosuppression: HIV infection of stem cells not allowing replenishment of T-cells; T-cells attacked (early) and loss of Th1 response (late)

HIV and Neurologic Disease

- crosses blood-brain barrier→invades glial cells→increases in brain cytokines (quinolinic acid, TGF-β→increases TNF-α→destroys neuronal cells→CNS disorders); damages neurons

GI Disease and Wasting

- multiplication in macrophages in lamina propria and enterochromaffin cells responsible for normal bowel motility and function

Cycle of Infection

- transmission of virus→infection of cell→replication→to lymph nodes→ replication→**HIV prodrome→vigorous immune response→clinical latency** lasting 5–10 years or more→low titer in blood but high in lymph nodes where CD4+ continues to decrease→ **opportunistic infections appear→** immune system collapse→degeneration of lymph nodes spills large amounts of virus into blood→progressive infection ensues

Clinical Course

- **seroconversion illness:** HIV prodrome or acute infection; resolve with HIV antibody formation
- **latency: patient infectious;** near end persistent generalized lymphadenopathy occurs; autoimmune disorders occur
- **symptomatic HIV infection with AIDS:** when CD4 count falls below 400/μm **AIDS-related complex begins→progression to AIDS→serious opportunistic infections; peripheral neuropathy; cancers; neurological disease (atrophy of cerebrum with sulci widening); inexorable wasting with diarrhea**

Diagnosis

- seroconversion illness: EIA for HIV p24/25 core antigen in blood is positive; HIV cultivation; positive PCR for viral nucleic acid; antibodies, cause circulation viral load to decrease
- latency: EIA for antibodies
- symptomatic infection: PCR can detect virus; decrease in CD4+ count and CD4+/CD8+ ratio decreases; if core antigen reappears prognosis is poor
- assessment of treatment: viral load and CD4+ count

Treatment

- goal to decrease viral burden by suppression of replication and prevent or treat opportunistic infection that arises

Dynamics of Infection

- **chance of drug-resistant mutant appearing even before therapy is high**
- goal of new therapy is to reach the level of <25 copies (viral RNA)/mL
- drug therapy should be considered long term
- antivirals: dideoxynucleoside analogues that inhibit RT: AZT, ddI, ddC, d4T, 3TC; non-nucleoside RT inhibitors: nevirapine; protease inhibitors: saquinavir, ritonavir, indinavir, nelfinavir
- combination therapy used: two RT inhibitors + protease inhibitor
- treatment of opportunistic infection: trimethoprim-sulfamethoxazole (TMP/SMX)

Principles of Infection

- always harmful; combination of drugs should always be used; measurement of HIV RNA levels and CD4+ cell counts necessary to follow disease and efficacy of treatment; women should receive optimal drug therapy regardless of pregnancy status; all patients infectious

Prevention

- no vaccine
- screen blood, body fluids, tissues for transplant
- individuals should be encouraged to change high-risk behavior

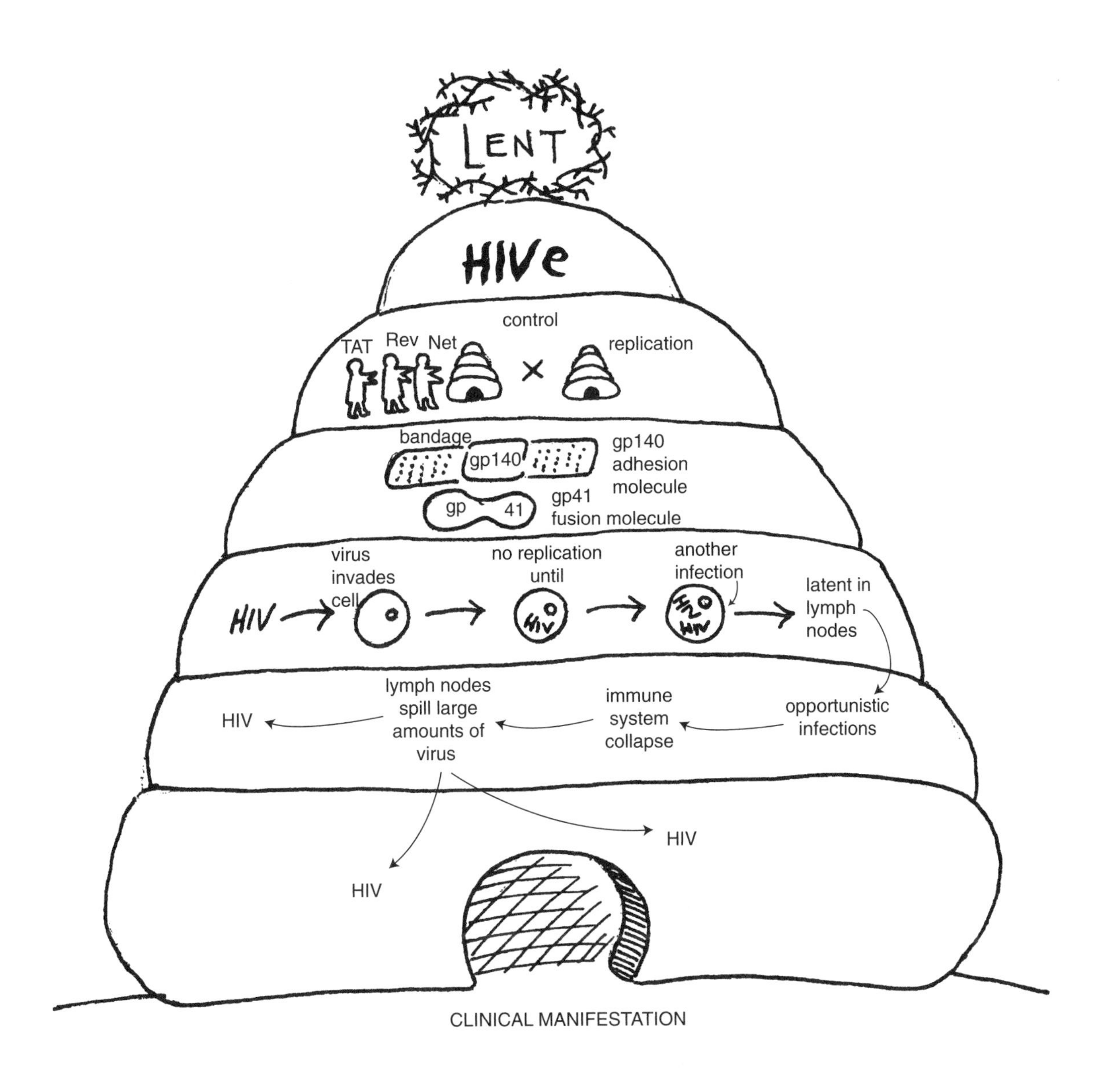

HIV neurological disease

HIV PRODROME

neurologic disease

GI wasting

HIV

AIDS

HIV

OPPORTUNISTIC

V.
IMMUNOLOGY

NOTES

AUTOIMMUNE DISORDERS

⇒ (auto + moon)

myasthenia gravis (gravity)

- anti-acetylcholine receptor antibody
- "STAY"—inability to transmit the Ach-induced signal; therefore signal stays

Sjögren's syndrome

- antibodies against salivary (Sally) duct antigens leading to dryness of mouth (sucker), trachea, bronchi, eyes, nose, vagina, and skin
- affects postmenopausal women (older women)

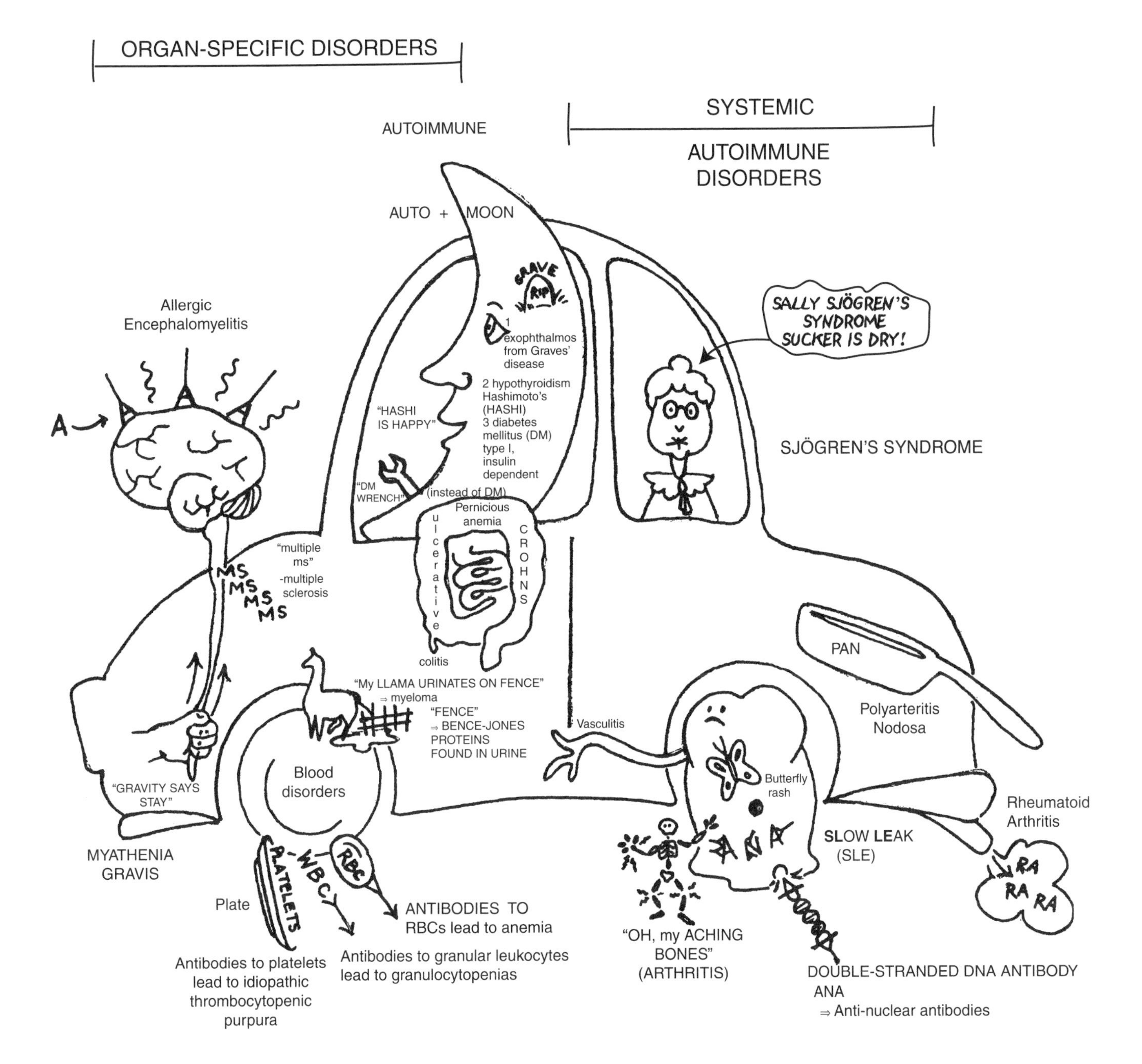
ORGAN-SPECIFIC DISORDERS
AUTOIMMUNE
SYSTEMIC
AUTOIMMUNE
DISORDERS
AUTO + MOON
GRAVE
RIP
1 exophthalmos from Graves' disease
2 hypothyroidism Hashimoto's (HASHI)
3 diabetes mellitus (DM) type I, insulin dependent
"HASHI IS HAPPY"
"DM WRENCH" (instead of DM)
Pernicious anemia
ulcerative colitis
CROHNS
SALLY SJÖGREN'S SYNDROME SUCKER IS DRY!
SJÖGREN'S SYNDROME
Allergic Encephalomyelitis
A
"multiple ms" -multiple sclerosis
MS MS MS MS
"My LLAMA URINATES ON FENCE" ⇒ myeloma
"FENCE" ⇒ BENCE-JONES PROTEINS FOUND IN URINE
Vasculitis
PAN
Polyarteritis Nodosa
"GRAVITY SAYS STAY"
MYATHENIA GRAVIS
Blood disorders
PLATELETS
WBC
RBC
Plate
ANTIBODIES TO RBCs lead to anemia
Antibodies to platelets lead to idiopathic thrombocytopenic purpura
Antibodies to granular leukocytes lead to granulocytopenias
Butterfly rash
ANA
SLOW LEAK (SLE)
Rheumatoid Arthritis
RA RA RA
"OH, my ACHING BONES" (ARTHRITIS)
DOUBLE-STRANDED DNA ANTIBODY
ANA
⇒ Anti-nuclear antibodies

NOTES

HYPERSENSITIVITIES

RA

⇒ rheumatoid arthritis

AR

⇒ Arthus reaction

PAN

⇒ polyarteritis nodosa

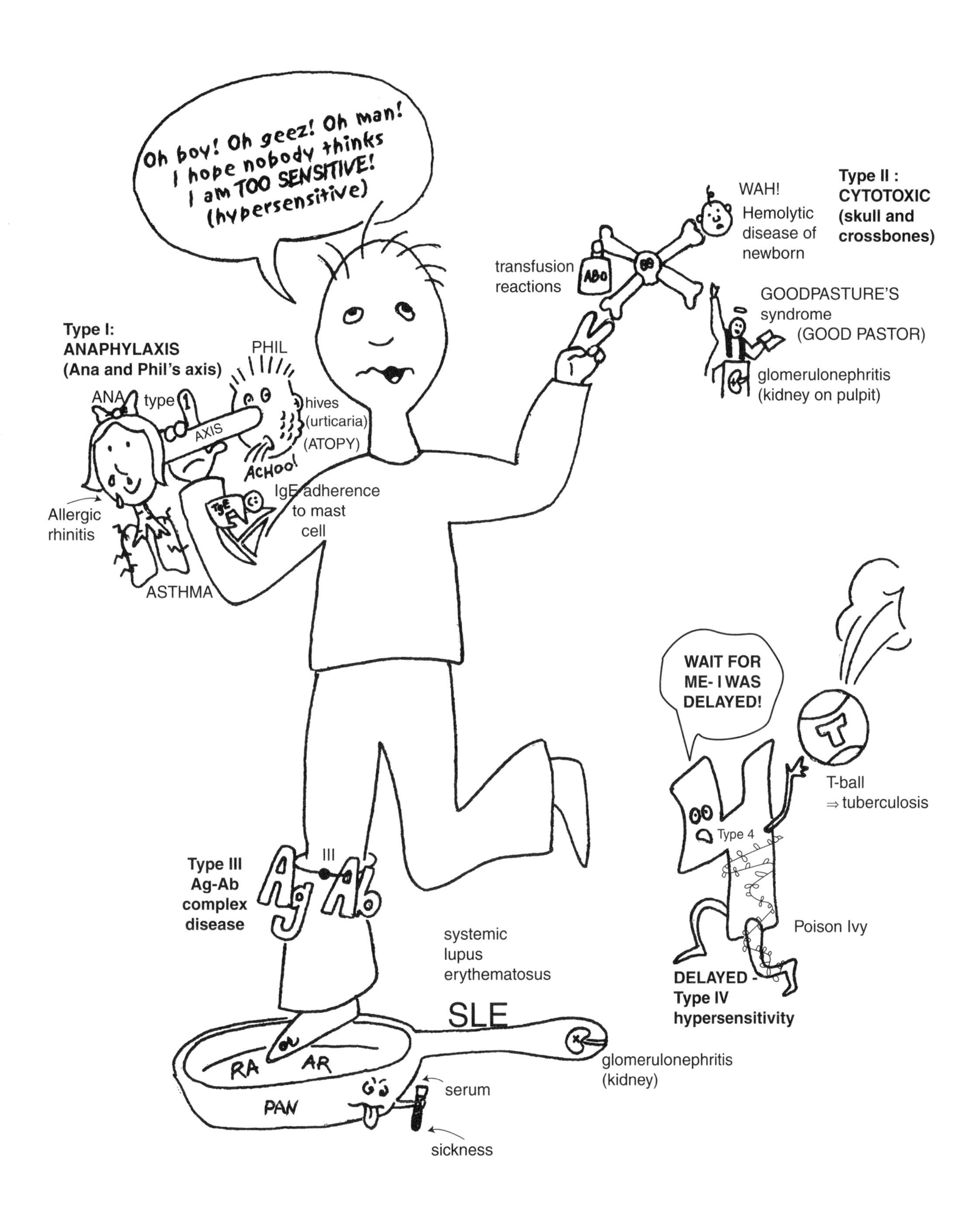
Oh boy! Oh geez! Oh man! I hope nobody thinks I am TOO SENSITIVE! (hypersensitive)
Type I: ANAPHYLAXIS (Ana and Phil's axis)
PHIL
ANA
type 1
AXIS
hives (urticaria) (ATOPY)
ACHOO!
IgE adherence to mast cell
IgE
Allergic rhinitis
ASTHMA
transfusion reactions
ABO
WAH!
Hemolytic disease of newborn
Type II : CYTOTOXIC (skull and crossbones)
GOODPASTURE'S syndrome (GOOD PASTOR)
glomerulonephritis (kidney on pulpit)
WAIT FOR ME- I WAS DELAYED!
T
T-ball ⇒ tuberculosis
Type 4
Poison Ivy
DELAYED - Type IV hypersensitivity
Type III Ag-Ab complex disease
III
Ag Ab
systemic lupus erythematosus
SLE
RA
AR
PAN
serum
sickness
glomerulonephritis (kidney)

INDEX